Table of Contents

Practice Test #1

Practice Questions

1. Outcomes assessment using small area analysis would be appropriate to determine
   [handwritten: method utilized to analyze variation in utilization of healthcare in small geographic or demographic areas]
   a. statewide hospital mortality rates.
   b. individual hospital utilization rates in a city. *(circled)*
   c. state-by-state comparisons of morbidity.
   d. statewide impact of reduction in Medicaid.

2. According to systems theory (von Bertalanffy), the element of a system that comprises actions that take place in order to transform input is
   a. throughput. *(circled)*
   b. output.
   c. evaluation.
   d. feedback.
   [handwritten: These are the 5 elements in a system]
   [handwritten: these are actions that take place to transform input]

3. Under provisions of the Family and Medical Leave Act (FMLA), how many workweeks of leave in a 12-month period is a worker entitled to in order to care for his son, an Army service member, who was seriously injured in a bombing incident?
   a. 10
   b. 12
   c. 26 *(circled)*
   d. 48
   [handwritten: Employee can take up to 26 weeks to care for family member c serious illness incurred in the line of duty on active duty]

4. Lean Six Sigma is a method that focuses process improvement on
   a. individual staff persons.
   b. short-term goals.
   c. individual projects. *(circled)*
   d. strategic goals.

5. In cost analysis, which of the following represents conformance costs?
   [handwritten: Costs related to preventing errors]
   a. Costs related to errors, failures, or defects, including duplications of service and malpractice
   b. All costs (processes, services, equipment, time, material, staff) necessary to provide products or processes without error
   c. Costs related to preventing errors, such as monitoring and evaluation *(circled)*
   d. Costs that are shared, such as infrastructure costs
   [handwritten: Non-conformance costs are related to errors, failures & defects.]

6. Which of the following terms is the legal element that refers to a failure to carry out duties in accordance with accepted and usual standards of practice?
   a. Duty
   b. Breach *(circled)*
   c. Causation
   d. Harm
   [handwritten: The 4 elements of malpractice]

- 4 -

7. When determining the burden of proof for acts of negligence related to malpractice, how would risk management classify willfully providing inadequate care while disregarding the safety and security of another?
    a. Negligent conduct
    b. Gross negligence
    c. Contributory negligence
    d. Comparative negligence

8. Which of the following methods is used to determine monetary savings resulting from planned interventions?
    a. Cost-benefit analysis → measures cost of event & intervention to demonstrate savings
    b. Cost-effective analysis → measures effectiveness of intervention
    c. Efficacy study
    d. Cost-utility analysis

9. A Medicare Advantage Plan (MAP) is a(n)
    a. supplemental (Medigap) insurance plan.
    b. form of Medicaid for Medicare recipients.
    c. optional plan administered by Medicare.
    d. plan approved by Medicare but administered by private insurance companies.

10. Which of the following could be defined as the commitment the organization is making to strategic planning?
    a. Vision statement – usually stated in a sentence or short paragraph
    b. Mission statement
    c. Goals
    d. Objectives

11. Which of the following actions is the best example of meaningful recognition as part of achieving a healthy work environment?
    a. Providing annual salary increases
    b. Providing salary increase with certification
    c. Telling a staff person who prevented a medical error that she demonstrated excellence in nursing
    d. Telling the board of directors that the hospital has an excellent staff

12. When instituting a plan for risk management, the primary concern in the statement of purpose should be
    a. reduction in financial risk.
    b. client safety. → should always be top priority
    c. decreased liability.
    d. scope of the program.

13. Which governmental agency is responsible for bloodborne pathogens standards? as well as other standards workplace
    a. CDC
    b. OSHA
    c. EPA
    d. FDA

14. With the continuous quality improvement (CQI) model, the focus of improvement is on which of the following?
    (a.) Organization and processes
    b. Staff
    c. Administrative personnel
    d. Clients

15. How soon after discharge must the Inpatient Rehabilitation Facility Patient Assessment Instrument (IRF-PAI) data on Medicare Part A fee-for-service or Medicare Part C (Advantage) patients be submitted to the CMS National Assessment Collection Database?
    a. Within 72 hours
    b. Within 7 days
    c. Within 17 days
    (d.) Within 27 days → 17 days + 10 day grace period

[handwritten margin note: - Pre-admit screening must be done in 48 hrs before admission - Rehab must complete post admission physical eval within 24 hrs of admission - POC must be documented within 4 days.]

16. What is the primary focus of workers' compensation?
    a. Prevent economic hardship
    (b.) Return people to work *[handwritten: - as quickly and safely as possible]*
    c. Contain costs
    d. Promote workers' safety

17. When fully implemented, the four domains associated with Hospital Value-Based Purchasing include (1) clinical process of care, (2) patient experience of care, (3) outcome mortality, and (4)
    a. documentation.
    b. re-hospitalization.
    (c.) efficiency.
    d. improvement.

18. Which ethical principle is involved when a worker who is pregnant is reassigned from a job that involves contact with teratogenic substances to a different job?
    (a.) Nonmaleficence
    b. Autonomy
    c. Beneficence
    d. Justice

19. The executive nurse determines that adequate staffing for a workplace location requires 160 hours per week for 52 weeks during the year. How many fulltime equivalent (FTE) staff persons are required?
    a. 2
    (b.) 4
    c. 8
    d. 16

20. Which of the following questions is appropriate to ask an applicant during an interview?
    a. "How many years ago did you finish college?"
    b. "Can you arrange day care for your child during work hours?"
    c. "Do you have any health problems?"
    (d.) "Can you provide an example of how you have dealt with issues of diversity at work?"

21. The nurse executive notes that one department in an organization has experienced a marked increase in accidents over the previous two-month period. What should the initial action be?

  a. Institute safety training for the department.
  b. Complete a worker survey.
  c. Evaluate all departmental changes.
  d. Recommend increased supervision.

22. The hospital uses electronic health records (EHRs) for employees and patients. Which type of data misuse occurs when the system allows a vendor to access private information?

  a. Security breach   ↳computer
  b. Identity theft
  c. Unauthorized access
  d. Privacy violation

23. Which type of budget is used to pay for general expenses, such as salary, education, insurance, and maintenance?

  a. Capital
  b. Operating
  c. Cash balance
  d. Master

24. Under the Affordable Care Act, an accountable care organization (ACO) is part of
  a. the mandated service delivery system.
  b. the private insurance initiative.
  c. Medicaid.
  d. the Medicare Shared Savings Program (MSSP).

Group of medical providers that accepts payments based on quality

25. Spend down is the process by which
  a. insurance companies pay benefits.
  b. insurance companies contract with stop-loss plans.
  c. people utilize funds in a health savings account.
  d. people spend down assets on medical bills to qualify for Medicaid.

people have too much income to qualify for medicaid. They may qualify for medicaid if they spend less income on medical bills.

26. The Health Insurance Portability and Accountability Act (HIPAA) mandates privacy and security rules (CFR, Title 45, Part 164) to ensure that health information and individual privacy is protected. Which of the following is part of the privacy rules?

  a. Protected information includes conversations between doctors and other healthcare providers. = privacy rule
  b. Any health information must be secure and protected against threats, hazards, or non-permitted disclosure. = security rule
  c. Implementation specifications must be addressed for any adopted standards.
  d. Access controls must include a unique identifier. = security requirement

27. New policies are being instituted based on evidence-based research, but some staff members are vocally resistant to the changes. What is the most appropriate action?
     a. Advise staff that complaining is counterproductive.
     b. Provide honest information about the reasons for the changes and how the changes will affect staff.
     c. Suggest that staff vote on whether to implement the changes.
     d. File a report with Human Resources about those complaining.

28. In evidence-based research, what do persistent erratic findings in tracking and trending suggest?
     a. Changes in patient population requiring changes in processes of care
     b. Errors in statistical analysis of processes of care
     c. Normal day-to-day variations in processes of care
     d. Processes of care inconsistent or inadequate

29. When gathering qualitative data, which of the following methods is most appropriate?
     a. Interview   ⤷ Researcher interpretation is important.
     b. Questionnaire
     c. Data mining
     d. Survey

30. Considering human subject protection, once a subject has agreed to participate in research, which of the following is an accurate statement?
     a. The subject may discontinue participation at any time.
     b. The subject must complete the research project.
     c. The subject must petition the Office of Human Research Protection to withdraw.
     d. The subject must give two weeks notice to withdraw.

31. If one of the healthcare facility's primary goals is to increase staff retention in order to meet the mission of providing excellent care, which of the following professional development activities should have priority?
     a. Development of web-based instruction modules
     b. Development of research activities
     c. Participation in state and local organizations
     d. Development of a mentoring program

32. The model of performance improvement that focuses on the needs of the customer is
     a. total quality management (TQM).
     b. continuous quality improvement (CQI).
     c. plan-do-study-act (PDSA).
     d. quality improvement process (QIP).

33. Pervasive leadership means that
     a. a strict hierarchical leadership model is utilized.
     b. leaders are developed and identified at all levels.
     c. the nurse executive is involved in all levels of decision making in the organization.
     d. a shared governance model is utilized.

34. Considering Tuckman's stages of group development, during which stage does the leader's input and direction decrease?
    a. Forming
    b. Storming
    c. Norming
    d. Performing

35. Under provisions of the Americans with Disabilities Act (1992), employers are allowed to ask applicants if they
    a. need work accommodations.
    b. have any type of disability.
    c. can carry out incidental functions of the job.
    d. will consent to a medical examination prior to a job offer.

36. The healthcare accreditation agency that assists purchasers of health plans and consumers to evaluate the performance of health plans is
    a. Centers for Medicare and Medicaid Services (CMS).
    b. TJC (formerly The Joint Commission).
    c. URAC.
    d. National Committee for Quality Assurance (NCQA).

37. In conducting research, which of the following types of studies represents one in which those with a condition (such as infection) are compared to those without the condition?
    a. Retrospective cohort study
    b. Prospective cohort study
    c. Case control study
    d. Cross-sectional study

38. For quality/performance improvement, the best tool to determine methods to streamline processes is
    a. root cause analysis.
    b. tracer methodology.
    c. family survey.
    d. staff survey.

39. The National Patient Safety Goals communication requirements related to telephone orders or reporting include
    a. the receiver "reading back" the orders or report.
    b. the receiver repeating each part of an order or report as it's given.
    c. the individual giving orders or reports asks if the information is understood.
    d. the individual giving orders or reports repeats each item twice.

40. The Agency for Healthcare Research and Quality's (AHRQ's) quality indicators (QI) that measure the quality of care for disorders sensitive to outpatient care (with good care reducing the need for hospitalization) are
    a. prevention QIs.
    b. inpatient QIs.
    c. patient safety indicators (PSIs).
    d. pediatric QIs.

- 9 -

41. The first step in negotiation for a nurse executive should be
    a. statement of problem.
    b. discussion.
    c. research.
    d. statement of financial limits.

42. In response to a recent increase in surgical site mortality rates in one hospital unit, which method is most indicated to determine the cause?
    a. External benchmarking
    b. Targeted surveillance
    c. Plan-do-check-act (PDCA)
    d. Root cause analysis

43. The state minimum wage is $1.00 higher than the federal minimum under the Fair Labor Standards Act (FLSA). When setting wages for staff at a small hospital with less than $500,000 in annual dollar volume, the nurse executive must
    a. comply with the federal minimum wage.
    b. comply with the state minimum wage.
    c. choose whether to comply with the Federal or state minimum.
    d. set wages independently as hospitals with less than $500,000 in annual dollar volume are exempt.

44. The pharmacy placed individual dosages of medication in an automatic dispensing cart with the right medicine but wrong dosage, and the nurse checked only the patient's name and name of the medication but failed to note the wrong dosage, resulting in a life-threatening overdose. In a just organizational culture, the correct response to the nurse is to
    a. suspend from duty.
    b. send for more training.
    c. terminate employment.
    d. console.

45. The nurse executive receives feedback during evaluation suggesting the staff feels the nurse is not accessible. Which of the following actions is likely to most effectively increase perceptions of accessibility?
    a. The nurse executive calls a staff meeting to discuss perceptions.
    b. The nurse executive sends out a memo advising staff to email concerns.
    c. The nurse executive schedules an open office hour weekly for staff to drop in.
    d. The nurse executive sends out a questionnaire to staff regarding concerns.

46. The first step in succession planning is to
    a. describe the behaviors, skills, and leadership qualities necessary for the role.
    b. develop an emergency plan.
    c. outline the needs of the organization.
    d. identify internal and/or external candidates.

47. The primary disadvantage of groupthink in an organization is that it
    a. disrupts harmony.
    b. stifles dissent.
    c. prevents focus on a single goal.
    d. interferes with implementation of new policies.

48. After implementing a new system at a cost of $100,000, the estimated profit at one year was $113,000. The return on investment (ROI) was
    a. 8.7%.
    Formula: Gain - Cost
    b. 0.087%.
    c. 13%.
    d. 1.3%.

49. Hospitals that receive Inpatient Prospective Payment System (IPPS) payments must complete how many Hospital Consumer Assessment of Healthcare Providers and Systems (HCAHPS) surveys over the four calendar quarters of a year?
    a. 100
    b. 200
    c. 300
    d. 400

50. Which of the following rights is included in the American Nurse Association's (ANA's) Bill of Rights for registered nurses?
    a. To go on strike for increased wages
    b. To work in a positive environment
    c. To be offered the chance for advancement
    d. To negotiate conditions of employment

51. When instituting an orientation program for a specific department that has experienced significant staff turnover, the nurse executive should first
    a. conduct literature research.
    b. complete a survey of needs.
    c. meet with the department administrator.
    d. review similar orientation programs.

52. The four factors that most motivate employees are (1) autonomy, (2) salary, (3) recognition, and (4)
    a. physical environment.
    b. respect.
    c. benefits.
    d. education.

53. Some staff members at a hospital want to join a union and plan to file an election petition with the National Labor Relations Board. How many employees must sign the petition before the NLRB takes action to facilitate an election?
    a. 60%
    b. 45%
    c. 30%
    d. 15%

54. The healthcare facility is considering upgrading the automatic medication dispensing carts, and the nurse executive has identified three potential vendors with whom to contract. In order to facilitate comparisons, the next step should be to
    a. network with others to determine which equipment they are using.
    b. conduct an Internet search for evaluations/comparisons.
    c. attend conference presentations by the vendors.
    d. send a Request for Information to the vendors.

55. The most persuasive argument for a nurse executive to take to a hospital board to request an increase in the ratio of professional nurses to patients is probably
    a. increased staff satisfaction.
    b. reduced overall costs.
    c. improved patient care.
    d. reduced staff turnover.

56. A nurse executive who believes in Douglas McGregor's Theory X, which states the average worker is unmotivated and does not care about the organization, will probably favor which type of organizational culture?
    a. Autocratic → makes decisions independently. Staff often feels left out.
    b. Democratic
    c. Bureaucratic
    d. Laissez-faire

57. A chart that shows the hierarchical system of the organization and relationships within that system is a(n)
    a. Ishikawa diagram.
    b. flow chart.
    c. Pareto diagram.
    d. organizational chart.

58. When considering crisis management to deal with internal or external disasters, which of the following is a reactive element as opposed to preventive?
    a. Establishing control barriers
    b. Direct observation and readiness activities
    c. Utilizing failure mode and effects analyses (FMEAs) for process design
    d. Root cause analysis of observed problem

59. Under the patient-centered medical home model of care, patient care is coordinated through a
    a. case manager.
    b. nurse practitioner.
    c. primary care physician.
    d. family member.

60. Which of the following provides privacy protection for healthcare organizations and members engaged in peer review activities?
    a. Health Insurance Portability and Accountability Act (HIPAA)
    b. The Joint Commission (TJC)
    c. Health Care Quality Improvement Act (HCQIA)
    d. Agency for Healthcare Research and Quality (AHRQ)

61. If a breach in privacy by a HIPAA-covered entity occurs and involves 200 patients, which of the following actions are required?
    a. Notify the individuals only within 60 days.
    b. Notify the individuals and provide notice to media outlets within 60 days.
    c. Notify the individuals, provide notice to media outlets, and notify the U.S. Department of Health and Human Services within 60 days. → >500 individuals
    d. Notify the individuals and notify the U.S. Department of Health and Human Services within 60 days of the end of the calendar year. → <500 individuals

62. A doctor offers the nurse executive a monetary reward for referring patients to his practice for Medicare reimbursable treatment. This is an example of violation of
    a. Health Insurance Portability and Accountability Act (HIPAA).
    b. Medicare and Medicaid Fraud and Abuse Law, Anti-Kickback Statute.
    c. Sarbanes-Oxley Act.
    d. Federal False Claims Act.

63. Which of the following is true about whistleblower protection? Whistleblowers are
    a. protected under one federal law.
    b. protected only under state law.
    c. protected under numerous federal and state laws.
    d. not protected by law.

64. In team-based nursing, the primary function of the team leader is
    a. delegation and supervision.
    b. documentation.
    c. direct patient care.
    d. communication with physicians.

65. Two 25-bed hospital units have the same scheduled nursing hours, but Unit A consistently requires three times more hours of overtime nursing than Unit B. To resolve this disparity, the nurse executive should first
    a. interview both unit administrators.
    b. recommend additional training for the administrator of Unit A.
    c. review acuity and census data for both units.
    d. review records of sick time, authorized, and unauthorized staff absences for both units.

66. Which three factors are considered when determining prices with the resource-based relative value scale (RBRVS) system?
    a. Physician work, patient diagnosis, and patient outcome
    b. Physician work, expense of practice, and expense of malpractice
    c. Physician work, patient diagnosis, and duration of care
    d. Physician work, patient outcome, and expense of practice

52% work
44% Practice
4% malpractice

67. In a hospital, the most critical factor in the revenue cycle is
    a. admission procedures.
    b. discharge procedures.
    c. collection of unpaid bills.
    d. patient outcomes.

68. If Medicare pays one payment to cover hospital and physician charges as well as charges of other practitioners for a hospitalized patient, this is an example of which type of bundling?
   a. Model 1: Retrospective Acute Care Hospital Stay Only
   b. Model 2: Retrospective Acute Care Hospital Stay plus Post-Acute Care
   c. Model 3: Retrospective Post-Acute Care Only
   d. Model 4: Acute Care Hospital Stay Only

69. If a registered nurse in an oncology unit believes that the team leader is working under the influence of drugs, the nurse should
   a. discuss suspicions with the team leader.
   b. report suspicions to the unit administrator.
   c. report suspicions to the board of directors.
   d. report suspicions to the nurse executive.

70. If purchasing $100,000 worth of new equipment with a useful life expectancy of five years and a salvage value of $10,000, using straight-line depreciation, what is the annual depreciation?
   a. $20,000
   b. $18,000
   c. $9,000
   d. $5,000

71. When using the Six Hats method of facilitating lateral thinking, wearing the red hat means
   a. examining facts and figures.
   b. making critical judgments.
   c. focusing on feelings.
   d. thinking creatively.

72. Operational budgets in which all cost centers are re-evaluated each budget period to determine if they should be funded or eliminated, partially or completely, are
   a. zero based.
   b. rolling.
   c. flexible.
   d. fixed/forecast.

73. In SWOT analysis, the S represents *strengths*, the W *weaknesses*, and the O *opportunities*. What does the T represent?
   a. Time
   b. Threats
   c. Targets
   d. Testing

74. Which category of evidence indicates that something is required by state or federal regulations or is an industry standard?
    a. IA
    b. IB
    c. IC
    d. II

75. When instituting a new and complex electronic medical record system in a large healthcare organization with multiple sites, the best approach is probably
    a. pilot implementation.
    b. parallel implementation.
    c. big-bang implementation.
    d. phased implementation.

76. When budgeting expenses, if the capital threshold is set at more than $600 and expected life span more than three years, which of the following would be considered a capital asset?
    a. Portable intravenous pole costing $120.00
    b. Portable ultrasound costing $18,000
    c. Dressing supplies costing $3000.00
    d. Instructional DVDs for the new electronic medical record system costing $500.00

77. Which of the following is an example of intelligent risk taking?
    a. Purchasing less expensive automatic medication dispensing carts for the entire facility without testing
    b. Decreasing ICU nursing hours by 20% to cut costs
    c. Announcing decreased benefits for all staff members
    d. Instituting new streamlined discharge procedure for one unit

78. Considering generational differences, which generation tends to be more reluctant to compromise if a conflict about different approaches to care arises?
    a. Silent generation (born before WWII)
    b. Baby Boomers (born 1943–1960)
    c. Generation X (born in the 1960s and 1970s)
    d. Millennial (Y) generation (born 1980–2000)

79. Which of the following methods of communicating performance measures is likely to be most effective if the nurse executive wants to reach and influence internal stakeholders?
    a. Digital dashboard, updated weekly
    b. Weekly print newsletter
    c. Monthly verbal reports at staff meetings
    d. Weekly briefings of all unit administrators

80. The nurse executive promotes development of a journal club to encourage staff members to
    a. write research articles.
    b. choose articles of interest to discuss.
    c. read and evaluate articles in scientific and professional journals.
    d. write personal journals expressing feelings and opinions.

81. When determining the skill mix for a specific hospital unit in order to increase the ratio of unlicensed assistive personnel as a cost-cutting measure, the most important factor for the nurse executive to consider is
    a. the grade of the professional nurses.
    b. the experience of the professional nurses.
    c. the experience of the unlicensed assistive personnel.
    d. the most cost-effective skill mix.

82. There are four primary core criteria for credentialing and privileging. The first three are licensure, education, and competence. What is the fourth?
    a. Performance ability
    b. Recommendations
    c. Currency of education
    d. Leadership

83. In order to facilitate quality improvement processes, the nurse executive should first
    a. build relationships among staff in order to facilitate change.
    b. delineate resource needs, including staffing and training, with a detailed budget.
    c. produce an internal action plan that describes problems that need resolution.
    d. secure support, resources, and approval from the governing board and key leaders.

84. Which of the following is an important element in coaching?
    a. Providing negative feedback, outlining the mistakes the person has made
    b. Using questioning to help the person recognize problem areas
    c. Asking the person to identify resources to help master material
    d. Providing a list of goals for the person to work toward

85. The nurse executive monitors national rates of hospital-acquired infections and compares them to internal rates. This is an example of
    a. internal trending.
    b. evidence-based research.
    c. external benchmarking.
    d. quality improvement.

86. The performance appraisal format should be primarily based on
    a. the person's job description.
    b. the skill level required for the position.
    c. departmental preference.
    d. readability level.

87. Which of the following is an example of shared governance?
    a. Unit teams establish work schedules for their own units
    b. Administrators receive regular reports of executive decisions
    c. The nurse executive allows incentive pay for 12-hour shifts
    d. Units are rewarded for achieving cost-cutting goals

88. When developing evidence-based practice guidelines, the first step is to
   a. conduct an evidence/literature review.
   b. consult experts.
   c. review policy considerations.
   d. focus on the topic and methodology.

89. The nurse executive is utilizing active listening when speaking with a staff member. Which of the following is the best statement to provide feedback to ensure the nurse executive understands the message of the staff member?
   a. "Do you want to be treated differently from other staff members?"
   b. "I can see that you are unhappy."
   c. "I understand you to say that you feel your working hours are excessive."
   d. "I don't understand what you are saying."

90. During a staff meeting, one member of the staff folds her arms across her chest and rolls her eyes while another staff member speaks about a problem he has encountered with the admission process. This is an example of
   a. sexual harassment.
   b. normal response to disagreement.
   c. horizontal violence.
   d. workplace discrimination.

91. When participating in the design of a new burn unit, the nurse executive states that the most important factor to consider is
   a. Infection control
   b. Staff preference
   c. Workflow
   d. Cost-effectiveness

92. When meeting with unit administrators, the nurse executive observes that the administrators have divided into two groups with conflicting opinions about an issue, and both sides are quite angry. The nurse executive should first
   a. encourage the administrators to discuss and resolve the issue.
   b. allow both sides to present their side of conflict without bias, maintaining a focus on opinions rather than individuals.
   c. force the two sides to reach a resolution.
   d. advise the groups that their behavior is unprofessional.

93. A Middle-Eastern patient in labor states that she does not want the male nurse to examine her during labor. The team leader reports to the administration that women in OB don't want to be cared for by male nurses. From a critical thinking perspective, this is an example of
   a. hasty generalization.
   b. overgeneralization.
   c. missing the point.
   d. appeal to ignorance.

94. The nurse executive notes that supply expenditures in one department routinely exceed budget allocation. Which problem-solving action is solution-focused as opposed to cause-focused?
    a. Review inventory procedures
    b. Discuss problem with unit administrator
    c. Increase supplies budget for the department
    d. Conduct a one-month study tracking supplies

95. When using the Shewhart cycle of plan-do-study-act (PDSA), *plan* usually begins with
    a. collecting data.
    b. identifying changes.
    c. generating solutions.
    d. brainstorming.

96. The most common method of determining patient satisfaction with care is to
    a. ask individual patients.
    b. provide discharge surveys.
    c. review patient complaints.
    d. ask staff members.

97. When scheduling a staff meeting, the most effective method for the nurse executive to employ is probably to
    a. place notices on bulletin boards.
    b. send an email notice.
    c. print a notice in the weekly organization newsletter.
    d. send reminders by regular mail.

98. The most effective method of hand-off of a patient from one department to another is to
    a. utilize the SBAR tool.
    b. consider critical information and report verbally.
    c. base hand-off report on receiver questions.
    d. prepare a brief written report.

99. In reflective communication, the ability to perceive the mental processes of the self and others is referred to as
    a. metacognition.
    b. mental telepathy.
    c. mindsight.
    d. mental focus.

100. Feedback is a critical element of which type of formal communication?
    a. Two-way communication
    b. One-way communication
    c. Public communication
    d. Nonverbal communication

101. Which of the following is an example of passive-aggressive communication?
   a. "I don't agree with this decision."
   b. "That's a ridiculous idea!"
   c. "Well, you're the boss, so I will do it your way."
   d. "I think there are better solutions to this problem."

102. The nurse executive is giving a report to the board of directors and must discuss financial issues and progress in quality improvement. Which of the following is probably the best communication method to use to facilitate understanding of the material?
   a. Video
   b. Handouts
   c. PowerPoint presentation
   d. Flip chart

103. Which of the following acts specifically states that adults have the right to refuse medical treatment?
   a. Americans with Disabilities Act
   b. Emergency Medical Treatment and Active Labor Act
   c. Patient Self-Determination Act— gives adults the right to refuse care.
   d. Older Americans Act

104. The practice model in which patients are placed in units according to their needs for care rather than their diagnosis so that all patients have similar needs for nursing is
   a. team nursing.
   b. case management.
   c. progressive patient care.
   d. primary care.

105. Which of the following is a specific multi-disciplinary care plan that outlines interventions and outcomes of diseases, conditions, and procedures?
   a. Flow sheet
   b. Clinical/critical pathway
   c. Standard protocol
   d. SOAP notes

106. Which of the following activities would probably preclude a patient from being classified as "homebound" for Medicare coverage of home health care?
   a. Patient's daughter takes the patient to religious services each week.
   b. Patient uses a walker to slowly ambulate about one-half block each day for exercise.
   c. Patient stays at an adult daycare center during weekdays while her caregiver works.
   d. Patient drives to a community college three days a week and takes classes in photography and painting.

107. The nurse executive wants to improve post-hospitalization healthcare management of COPD patients in order to reduce re-hospitalization. Which of the following is the best targeted approach?

a. Posters about COPD are placed in clinics and doctors' offices.

b. A series of one-hour classes are scheduled to teach 15 to 20 COPD patients about disease management.

c. The nurse executive appears on a local TV health program to discuss care for COPD.

d. Patients are provided booklets about COPD care on discharge.

108. The Joint Commission's ORXY requirement for data for freestanding children's hospitals is

a. three core measures (including Children's Asthma Care) and three non-core measures.

b. one core measure (Children's Asthma Care) and nine non-core measures.

c. four core measures, including Children's Asthma Care.

d. nine non-core measures only.

*most core measures are related to adults → see core measures list on pg 45.

109. Which of the following must be treated as a sentinel event?

a. A patient with metastatic liver cancer dies.

b. A patient with ALS dies from pneumonia.

c. A discharged patient dies from an intentional overdose of prescribed pain medications.

d. A surgeon operates on the wrong knee.

↳ deaths or serious injuries that are unexpected.

110. Which of the following is a key element for a healthy work environment?

a. Consistent models of care

b. High salaries

c. Patient advocacy

d. Meaningful recognition

111. According to the Joint Commission's leadership standards, who has ultimate responsibility for all patient care within the jurisdiction of the organization?

a. Chief executive officer

b. Chief medical officer

c. Governing board

d. Nurse executive

112. Which of the following is an example of a back-end e-health exchange of data?

a. A patient emails a question to a physician.

b. A patient sends a picture of a wound to a physician.

c. The physician responds to a patient email.

d. The physician requests a patient's medical records from a previous physician.

113. A time-limited arrangement that can involve shared care or direct supervision, related to a term of study, such as a semester, is

a. mentoring.

b. coaching.

c. precepting.

d. training.

114. The ability to look at a person's facial expression and to understand and perceive that person's emotions is an element of
    a. emotional intelligence.
    b. intellectual ability.
    c. body language comprehension.
    d. facial recognition.

115. The nurse executive is concerned at the high turnover rate of nurses in the oncology unit because of job stress. Which intervention is most likely to aid retention?
    a. Formation of a peer support group
    b. Referral of staff to psychologists
    c. Inservice on dealing with stress
    d. Coaching

116. When creating a pro forma business plan, which of the following is the most important element?
    a. Business aims
    b. Business objectives
    c. Business market
    d. Business activity

117. Servant leadership suggests that
    a. all staff members of the organization serve the leader.
    b. the leader serves all others in the organization.
    c. a hierarchical system of leadership is in place.
    d. staff members are assigned specific tasks to assist the leader.

118. Corporate compliance means
    a. ensuring that controls are in place to prevent violations of rules, laws, and regulations.
    b. following the directions of the board of directors.
    c. complying with industry standards.
    d. establishing a governing board.

119. Which of the following is an example of a push strategy for knowledge management?
    a. Creating a database of shared knowledge
    b. Storytelling
    c. Experts sharing information directly
    d. Knowledge fair

120. Which is the most critical element in creating a culture of staff accountability?
    a. Performance measures
    b. Leadership
    c. Infrastructure support
    d. Resources

121. The most important reason for the nurse executive to take continuing education courses is to
   a. maintain and improve professional skills.
   b. find networking opportunities.
   c. set a good example for staff.
   d. meet job requirements.

122. The nurse executive is addressing a staff member who averts her eyes and avoids direct eye contact. The nurse executive should assume that
   a. the person is lying.
   b. the person is shy.
   c. the person is afraid of the nurse executive.
   d. no assumption about the person can be made without further information.

123. Which type of facility requires that a patient need and be prescribed at least three hours of a minimum of two types of therapy daily?
   a. Skilled nursing facility
   b. Inpatient rehabilitation facility
   c. Ambulatory care center
   d. Critical care hospital

124. With win-win negotiating, the critical factor the nurse executive should go to negotiations knowing is
   a. the potential settlement area.
   b. the other negotiator's needs/demands.
   c. the time frame for negotiations.
   d. the desired outcome.

125. The nurse executive has received four different complaints about the rude behavior of one of the program directors toward staff members. The most appropriate way to initially address concerns with the director is at a
   a. board meeting.
   b. staff meeting.
   c. one-on-one conversation.
   d. disciplinary hearing.

126. The primary role of a patient/family advisory council is to
   a. address the needs of patients/families.
   b. establish new procedures.
   c. make policies.
   d. outline deficiencies in care.

127. Which of the following statements exemplifies an assertive communication style when faced with a person providing an unworkable solution to a problem?
   a. "That's a ridiculous idea!"
   b. "I'm not sure that will work, but I guess we can try."
   c. "That's an interesting idea, but here are the problems…."
   d. "You should know that won't work."

128. Considering the clinical quality measures (CQM) for the CMS electronic health record incentive programs (2014), to which domain does the CQM "Weight Assessment and Counseling for Nutrition and Physical Activity for Children and Adolescents" belong?
a. Efficient use of healthcare resources
b. Population/public health
c. Patient and family engagement
d. Patient safety

129. In a customer service model that stresses service recovery, what is the first step to take when a mistake has occurred?
a. Provide compensation
b. Apologize
c. Make an excuse
d. Deny the mistake occurred

130. One of the most effective ways to network is to
a. email colleagues.
b. utilize LinkedIn or Facebook.
c. meet regularly with colleagues.
d. become involved in national organizations and conferences.

131. The nurse executive uses the STAR method to increase visibility and share success in program improvement. The STAR method comprises:
a. situation, task, action, results.
b. start, timetable, action, recommendations.
c. site, time, achievement, reaction.
d. situation, timetable, action, reaction.

132. Which of the following is the most significant barrier to development of a culture of transparency to improve patient safety?
a. Lack of knowledge
b. Inadequate leadership
c. Staff resistance
d. Fear of punitive action or retribution

133. A balanced scorecard should be based primarily on the
a. goals and objectives.
b. mission statement.
c. vision statement.
d. strategic plan.

134. When reviewing the types of data required for strategic planning, an example of aggregate data is data regarding
a. hazard and safety practices.
b. library services or access to information.
c. benchmarks.
d. informed consent.

Copyright © Mometrix Media. You have been licensed one copy of this document for personal use only. Any other reproduction or redistribution is strictly prohibited. All rights reserved.

135. Under the Affordable Care Act (ACA), which of the following is part of the new Patient's Bill of Rights?
    a. Insurance companies may not retroactively cancel the policy of a patient who becomes ill.
    b. Health plans must explicitly state if they cover or exclude children.
    c. All health plans must immediately eliminate all annual compensation limits.
    d. Out-of-network providers cannot send bills for service (balanced billing) not covered by the health plan.

136. When establishing baseline data, what period of time for surveillance and review is typically used?
    a. One week
    b. Two weeks
    c. One month
    d. Two months

137. Which of the following states clearly that the nurse's primary commitment is to the patient?
    a. Affordable Care Patient's Bill of Rights
    b. ANA Code of Ethics
    c. AMA Code of Medical Ethics
    d. Code of Ethics and Standards of Practice for Healthcare Professionals

138. The primary responsibility of a bioethics committee is to
    a. resolve conflicts between staff members.
    b. evaluate reports of negligence.
    c. educate staff about ethics.
    d. determine the most morally correct action given the circumstances.

139. The primary purpose in establishing a performance improvement team is to
    a. improve cost effectiveness.
    b. improve outcomes through common purpose.
    c. promote staff cooperation.
    d. meet regulatory requirements.

140. When measuring performance, which of the following may be defined as an external trigger to signal the need for further analysis?
    a. Rate changes
    b. Sentinel events
    c. Benchmarks
    d. Performance rate

141. Which of the following statements is a violation of informed consent when a patient who is signing a consent form for chemotherapy asks what adverse effects to expect from the chemotherapeutic agent?
    a. "About 8 in 10 patients experience nausea and vomiting."
    b. "You don't need to worry about that. You will receive medications to control the adverse effects."
    c. "I don't know, but I will get that information for you before you sign."
    d. "Let's go over this pamphlet outlining side effects together."

142. Because of concerns about mortality rates, the hospital has collected data which shows a ranking of physicians from those with the highest mortality rates to those with the lowest. This information about ranking should be provided to
    a. all staff members.
    b. all medical staff members.
    c. the individual physicians.
    d. all administrative staff.

143. The four Ds of appreciative inquiry are (1) discover, (2) dream, (3) design and (4)
    a. discard/disallow.
    b. differentiate.
    c. display.
    d. destiny/deliver.

144. Which trend has had the greatest impact on healthcare in the last 10 to 20 years?
    a. Technological advances
    b. Aging population
    c. Economic globalization
    d. Educated consumers

145. The theory of leadership that states that there is no best method of leadership but that a leader's skill must match the needs of the situation is
    a. trait theory.
    b. contingency theory.
    c. skills theory.
    d. transformation theory.

146. Which government agency requires that healthcare facilities file semiannual reports regarding problems with drugs or equipment to the website MedWatch?
    a. OSHA
    b. FDA
    c. CDC
    d. CMS

147. Which of the following is responsible for screening patients from the time of admission (or before admission in some cases) and assisting with planning for discharge?
    a. Physician
    b. Unit administrator
    c. Nurse executive
    d. Case manager

148. In order to avoid potential biases related to cultural differences, which of the following is essential for the nurse executive?
    a. Experience with various cultures
    b. Diversity training
    c. Knowledge of laws related to discrimination
    d. Self-awareness

149. When conducting research, the first step in critical reading is to
    a. examine the article organization.
    b. determine the thesis.
    c. review the article's evidence.
    d. consider the source of the material.

150. Before beginning a grant application process, the nurse executive should
    a. establish a timeline.
    b. provide a detailed budget.
    c. collect preliminary data.
    d. complete the literature review.

$$\begin{array}{r} 150 \\ -\ 44 \\ \hline 106 \end{array}$$

$$\frac{106}{150} = 70.0\%$$

Answers and Explanations

1. B: Outcomes assessment of large areas, such as counties or states, merges data so that the results often reflect averages that don't accurately reflect the reality in small areas. Small area analysis is appropriate to look at data in a prescribed "small" area, such as determining rates of hospital utilization at individual hospitals rather than compiling that information into one statistical average, because there may be pronounced statistical differences that have been overlooked. Small area analysis is most often applied to epidemiologic data and rates of hospital utilization.

2. A: Throughput. The five elements in a system include:
- Input: This is what goes into a system in terms of energy or materials.
- Throughput: These are the actions that take place in order to transform input.
- Output: This is the result of the interrelationship between input and processes.
- Evaluation: This is the process of monitoring success or failure.
- Feedback: This is information that results from the process and can be used to evaluate the end result.

Bertalanffy believed that all of the elements of a system interact in order to achieve goals, and change in any one element will impact the other elements and alter outcomes.

3. C: FMLA allows 26 workweeks of leave in a 12-month period to provide care to a military service member who is a spouse, child, parent, or next of kin as part of military caregiver leave. Other entitlements include 12 workweeks of leave in a 12-month period for the birth of a child, adoption or foster care of a child (newly placed), illness of spouse, child, or parent, and a health condition that interferes with the ability to carry out job functions.

4. D: Lean Six Sigma combines Six Sigma with concepts of "lean" thinking, focusing process improvement on strategic goals rather than on a project-by-project basis. This type of program is driven by strong senior leadership that outlines long-term goals and strategies. The basis is to reduce error and waste within the organization through continuous learning and rapid change. Characteristics include:
- Long-term goals with strategies in place for one- to three-year periods.
- Performance improvement as the underlying belief system.
- Cost reduction through quality increase, supported by statistics evaluating the cost of inefficiency.
- Incorporation of improvement methodology (such as PDSA).

5. C: Conformance costs include those related to preventing errors, such as monitoring and evaluation. Nonconformance costs are those related to errors, failures, and defects. These may include adverse events (such as infections), poor access due to staff shortages or cancellations, lost time, duplications of service, and malpractice. Error-free costs are all those costs in terms of processes, services, equipment, time, materials, and staffing that are necessary to providing a product or process that is without error from the onset. Indirect costs are shared costs, such as infrastructure costs and the cost of custodial services.

6. B: Breach is the legal element of negligence that refers to a failure to carry out duties in accordance with accepted and usual standards of practice. Duty is a legal responsibility or obligation that relates to a relationship (such as parent to protect his/her child) or statute (such as the requirement for a nurse to report child abuse). Causation is the direct proof that a breach of duty resulted in harm. Harm is the injury that results from a breach of duty.

7. B: Gross negligence. Negligence indicates that *proper care* has not been provided, based on established standards. *Reasonable care* uses rationale for decision making in relation to providing care. Types of negligence include:
- Negligent conduct indicates that an individual failed to provide reasonable care or to protect/assist another, based on standards and expertise.
- Gross negligence is willfully providing inadequate care while disregarding the safety and security of another.
- Contributory negligence involves the injured party contributing to his/her own harm.
- Comparative negligence attempts to determine what percentage amount of negligence is attributed to each individual involved.

8. A: A cost-benefit analysis uses average cost of an event and the cost of intervention to demonstrate savings. A cost-effective analysis measures the effectiveness of an intervention rather than the monetary savings. Efficacy studies may compare a series of cost-benefit analyses to determine the intervention with the best cost-benefit. They may also be used for process or product evaluation. Cost-utility analysis (CUA) is essentially a sub-type of cost-effective analysis, but it is more complex and the results are more difficult to quantify and use to justify expense because cost-utility analysis measures benefit to society in general, such as by decreasing teen pregnancy.

9. D: A Medicare Advantage Plan (MAP) is approved by Medicare but administered by private insurance companies. These plans must follow the rules established by Medicare. Medicare pays a fixed amount per month to the insurance company for beneficiaries who are enrolled. A MAP is a form of managed care, so while all of the services provided under Medicare A and B are covered, the MAP may offer additional services, such as dental and vision care, but offers less flexibility as healthcare providers must be chosen from a network and preapproval is required for treatment.

10. A: The vision statement is the commitment that the organization is making to strategic planning. The vision statement should include future goals rather than focusing on what has already been achieved. The vision statement is usually stated in a sentence or short paragraph:
> Hospital X will be the leader in providing sustainable quality patient-centered care to the community to improve the physical and mental health of community members.

The vision statement is often followed by an explanation of terms, so that such concepts as "sustainable" and "patient-centered" are clarified to explain the reason for including the terms in the vision statement.

11. C: While providing financial incentives (such as salary increases for certification) are one way to show recognition, they tend to be triggered automatically, so the best example of meaningful recognition is telling a staff person who prevented a medical error that she demonstrated excellence in nursing because this recognizes a real contribution and provides feedback on an individual basis. Some hospitals nominate nurses and other

caregivers as "caregiver of the month" or a similar form of recognition, but positive feedback should be done on a daily basis as well as a focus of leadership.

12. B: Client safety should always be the primary concern for risk management. Reduction of financial risks and liability relate directly to client safety. A risk management plan should include:
- Goals: Specific and measurable.
- Program scope: Should include linkage with other programs.
- Line of authority: Beginning with the governing board and ending with employees.
- Policies: Should include confidentiality and conflict of interest.
- Data sources and referrals: Types of measures.
- Documentation/reporting: The responsibility for reporting should be clarified as well as the frequency of reports.
- Activities integration.
- Evaluation of program: The method and frequency of evaluation.
- Charts/Diagrams: Flow charts, organizational charts, and diagrams.

13. B: OSHA, under the Department of Labor, is responsible for bloodborne pathogens standards as well as other workplace standards and inspection of workplaces to ensure safety standards are met. The CDC provides treatment guidelines and recommendations and monitors public health, compiling statistics regarding reportable disease. The EPA is not a statutory agency but provides information about the environment to other governmental agencies. The FDA is a consumer protection agency ensuring safety of medications, biological products, medical devices, and food.

14. A: CQI emphasizes the organization, systems, and processes within that organization rather than individuals. It recognizes internal customers (staff) and external customers (clients) and utilizes data to improve processes, recognizing that most processes can be improved. CQI uses the scientific method of experimentation to meet needs and improve services and utilizes various tools, such as brainstorming, multivoting, various charts and diagrams, storyboarding, and meetings. Core concepts include the following:
- Quality and success is meeting or exceeding internal and external customer's needs and expectations.
- Problems relate to processes, and variations in process lead to variations in results.
- Change can be incremental.

15. D: The IRF-PAI data on Medicare Part A FFS or Medicare Part C (Advantage) must be submitted to the CMS National Assessment Collection Database within 27 days (17 days plus a 10-day grace period). Required documents in the medical records include the preadmission screening to ascertain patient eligibility. This must be completed within the 48 hours prior to admission. If done before 48 hours, it must be repeated. The rehabilitation physician must complete a post-admission physical evaluation within 24 hours of admission. The admission orders must be written at the time of admission and the individual plan of care within four days.

16. B: The primary focus of worker's compensation, a type of insurance, is to return people to work as quickly and safely as possible. Worker's compensation is intended for those who are injured on the job or whose health is impaired because of their jobs. Worker's compensation provides three different types of benefits: cash to replace lost wages,

reimbursement for medical costs associated with the injury, and death benefits to survivors. Worker's compensation laws may vary somewhat from one state to another.

17. C: The four domains associated with Hospital Value-Based Purchasing include (1) clinical process of care, (2) patient experience of care, (3) outcome mortality, and (4) efficiency. Hospital Value-Based Purchasing reimburses hospitals based on quality of care and is being implemented in three phases, beginning in 2013 and to be completed by 2015. In 2013, clinical process is weighted at 70% and patient experience at 30%. In 2014, the weighting changes to clinical processes 45%, patient experience 30%, and outcome 25%. When fully implemented, the weight again changes to clinical 20%, patient experience 30%, outcome 30% and efficiency 20%.

18. A: Nonmaleficence is an ethical principle that means an employer should prevent intentional harm to the worker, such as by reassigning a pregnant worker to a job that does not endanger the fetus. Beneficence is the ethical principle that involves performing actions that are for the purpose of benefitting another person. Autonomy is the ethical principle that the individual has the right to make decisions about his/her own work. Justice is the ethical principle that relates to the distribution of the limited resources.

19. B: Four fulltime equivalent (FTE) staff persons are required. The formula for calculating fulltime equivalent (FTE) staffing helps to determine staffing needs:
- 40 hr/wk x 52 wk/yr = 1 FTE.
- 160 hr/wk x 52 wk/yr = 4 FTE.
- 20 hr/wk x 52 wk/yr = 0.5 FTE.

Staffing must include coverage/policies for break and meal times. Staffing includes both daytime hours and nighttime. Workplaces vary in shift duration: five 8-hour shifts, four 10-hour shifts, or three 12-hour shifts, but overtime pay may be a consideration with longer shifts.

20. D: An appropriate interview question is "Can you provide an example of how you have dealt with issues of diversity at work?" because it relates to performance. The nurse executive should avoid asking questions that may be interpreted as age discrimination, such as questions about when a person finished college, or personal/family questions, such as about caring for children, as these are not job-related and may suggest bias. The nurse executive can ask applicants if they need work accommodations but not if they have health problems.

21. C: The initial action should be to evaluate all departmental changes that have occurred and may have resulted in more accidents. This may include new staff, changes in equipment, or different procedures. This information coupled with data about the types of injuries may help the nurse executive to focus on the cause of the problem and arrive at the best solution, which may include altering processes or changing equipment, instituting safety training, doing job-specific training, conducting surveys, providing assistive devices, or increasing supervision.

22. A: Security breach: Careless or inadequate security allows others, such as billing companies or vendors, to have access to private information. Identity theft: Someone obtains identifying information, such as Social Security numbers and credit card numbers as well as birthdates and addresses, for fraudulent purposes. Unauthorized access: Although EHRs and computerized documentation systems are password protected, providers

sometimes share passwords or unwittingly expose their passwords to others when logging in, allowing others to access information about patients. Privacy violations: Even those authorized to access a patient's record may share private information with others, such as family or friends.

23. B: Operating budget: Used for daily operations and includes general expenses, such as salaries, education, insurance, maintenance, depreciation, debts, and profit. The budget has three elements: statistics, expenses, and revenue. Capital budget: Determines which capital projects (such as remodeling, repairing, purchasing of equipment or buildings) will be allocated funding for the year. These capital expenditures are usually based on cost-benefit analysis and prioritization of needs. Cash balance budget: Projects cash balances for a specific future time period, including all operating and capital budget items. Master budget: Combines operating, capital, and cash balance budgets as well as any specialized or area-specific budgets.

24. D: Under the Affordable Care Act, an Accountable Care Organization (ACO) is part of a Medicare Shared Savings Program (MSSP), in which volunteer groups of physicians and other healthcare providers and medical facilities form an organization to provide and coordinate care to groups of beneficiaries (minimum 5000) in return for financial incentives. The ACO must participate for a minimum of three years and must institute quality measures and cost-containment strategies. The ACO receives a percentage of savings, based on benchmark levels.

25. D: Spend down is the process by which people spend down assets on medical bills to qualify for Medicaid. Medicaid is administered by states, so regulations vary, but in order to qualify, people must be low income. However, if they have no or inadequate insurance, they can deduct the costs (paid or unpaid bills) they have incurred for medical services from their excess income in order to qualify. Once the spend down reaches the income requirement, Medicaid will pay the remaining medical bills.

26. A: Privacy rule: Protected information includes any information included in the medical record, conversations between the doctor and other healthcare providers, billing information, and any other form of health information. Security rule: Any electronic health information must be secure and protected against threats, hazards, or non-permitted disclosures. Implementation specifications must be addressed for any adopted standards. Security requirements include limiting access to those authorized, use of unique identifiers for each user, automatic logoff, encryption and decryption of protected healthcare information, authentication that healthcare data has not been altered/destroyed, monitoring of logins, authentication, and security of transmission.

27. B: When instituting changes, the best approach is to provide honest information about the reasons for changes and how staff will be affected. Resistance to change is common for many people, so coordinating collaborative processes requires anticipating resistance and taking steps to achieve cooperation. Resistance often relates to concerns about job loss, increased responsibilities, and general denial or lack of understanding and frustration. The nurse executive should be empathetic but assertive.

28. D: While trends will show some normal variation, if the trend becomes erratic and measures are inconsistent, this suggests that the processes of care are not consistent or are inadequate. Tracking and trending is central to developing research-supported evidence-

based practice and is part of continuous quality improvement. Once processes and outcomes measurements are selected, then at least one measure should be tracked for a number of periods of time, usually in increments of four weeks or quarterly. This tracking can be used to present graphical representation of results that will show trends.

29. A: Qualitative data are described verbally or graphically, and the results are subjective. Interviews may be used as a tool to gather information, and the researcher's interpretation of data is important. Gathering this type of data can be time-intensive, and it can usually not be generalized to a larger population.
Quantitative data are described in terms of numbers within a statistical format. This type of information gathering is done after the design of data collection is outlined, usually in later stages. Tools may include surveys, questionnaires, or other methods of obtaining numerical data. The researcher's role is objective.

30. A: Participation is voluntary and the subject can discontinue participation at any time without penalty. Risks should be minimal, and selection of subjects should be equitable. Any researcher involving patients in research must obtain informed consent, in language understandable to the patient or the patient's agent. The elements of this informed consent must include an explanation of the research, the purpose, and the expected duration as well as a description of any potential risks. Potential benefits must be described as well as possible alternative treatments. Any compensation to be provided must be outlined. The extent of confidentiality should be clarified.

31. D: Establishing a mentoring program is directly tied to the goal and mission statement and should have priority. Mentoring occurs in many different ways. A nurse may establish one-on-one mentoring relationships, but just as often taking the time to assist others on a one-time basis or working with groups of staff provides an opportunity for mentoring. Mentoring is a reciprocal activity because both mentor and the mentee benefit. Mentoring is central to the role of the CNS and can be incorporated into current practice without involving extensive added responsibilities or time commitments.

32. A: TQM is a philosophy of quality management that espouses a commitment to meeting the needs of the customers at all levels within an organization. CQI emphasizes the organization and systems and processes within that organization rather than individuals. PDSA is a method of continuous quality improvement. PDSA is simple and understandable; however, it may be difficult to maintain this cycle consistently because of lack of focus and commitment. QIP is a four-step method, focusing on quality control, which is based on a trilogy of concepts that include quality planning, control, and improvement.

33. B: Pervasive leadership recognizes that there are effective leaders at all levels in an organization and develops, nurtures, and identifies those leaders, encouraging their input into decision making and policies rather than imposing decisions from the top down. Organizations practicing pervasive leadership realize that leadership is often a learned skill and provide opportunities through coaching, mentoring, and training for people to assume increasing leadership roles. Pervasive leadership expressly recognizes the contributions of all members of an organization, helping to improve staff morale and commitment to the organization.

34. D: Performing. Tuckman's stages include:
- Forming: The leader lists the goals and rules and encourages communication.

- Storming: A divergence of opinions regarding management, power, and authority may lead to increased stress and resistance with absence of members, shared silence, and subgroup formation.
- Norming: Members express positive feelings toward each other and feel deeply attached to the group.
- Performing: The leader's input and direction decreases and mainly consists of keeping the group on course.
- Mourning: This is most deeply felt in closed groups when discontinuation of the group nears and in open groups when the leader or other members leave.

35. A: The ADA provides the disabled, including those with mental impairment, access to employment and the community. Employers are only allowed to ask applicants if they need accommodations, not if they have disabilities. Applicants may be asked if they can carry out essential functions of a job, not incidental functions, and medical examinations can only be required after a job is offered. Accommodations can include alterations in work station, speech recognition software, screen magnifying software, optical character recognition systems, video captioning, Braille readers and screen readers, adapted keyboards and on-screen keyboard, TTYs (text telephones), and amplification systems.

36. D: NCQA administers the Healthcare Effectiveness Data and Information Set (HEDIS) to measure performance of healthcare plans and to help identify plans that provide competent care. NCAQ collects data to demonstrate comparability and consistency in various health plans. Accreditation categories include quality improvement, physician credentials, members' rights/responsibilities, preventive services, utilization management, and medical records. HEDIS categories include effectiveness of care, accessibility and availability of care, satisfaction, cost of care, informed decision making, use of services, plan description, and health plan stability.

37. C: Case control studies compare those with a condition (cases) to a group without (controls) to determine if the affected group has characteristics that are different. Prospective cohort studies choose a group of patients without disease, assess risk factors, and then follow the group over time to determine (prospect for) which ones develop disease. Retrospective cohort studies are initiated after a condition develops and data is collected retrospectively from medical records to evaluate whether members of the cohort selected had exposure and developed disease. Cross-sectional studies assess both disease and exposure at the same time in a target population, evaluating the presence of disease at a point in time.

38. B: Tracer methodology looks at the continuum of care a client receives from admission to post-discharge. A client is selected to be "traced" and the medical record serves as a guide. Tracer methodology uses the experience of this client to evaluate the processes in place through documents and interviews. Root cause analysis (RCA) is a retrospective attempt to determine the cause of an event, or a cluster of events. Family and staff surveys may provide helpful but less detailed information.

39. A: The NPSG's requirement for telephone orders or reporting requires that after the information is received and documented, the receiver "read back" the information to ensure that it was heard and documented correctly. Other communication requirements include using a list of approved abbreviations and avoiding unclear or ambiguous abbreviations, acronyms, symbols, or dose designations. Reporting should be done in a timely manner, and

the organization should have a standardized manner of hand-off communication that allows for a time to ask/answer questions.

40. A: Prevention QIs measure the quality of care for disorders (such as diabetes and heart disease) sensitive to outpatient care, with good care reducing the risk of complications and the need for hospitalization. Inpatient QIs measure the quality of care within a hospital and include morbidity and mortality rates for different disorders, utilization of procedures, and volumes of procedures. PSIs measure complications and adverse events in hospitals related to surgery, procedures, and labor and delivery. Pediatric QIs measures adverse effects of healthcare exposure in the pediatric population.

41. C: The first step in negotiation for a nurse executive should be research to determine current market values and utilization. The nurse executive must go to negotiations prepared with facts and figures. Aggressively starting with financial limits or demands about costs is counterproductive, especially if they are unrealistic. Once research is completed, then the nurse executive can give a statement of the problem and the elements needed to solve the problem. Clear, honest, open communication is essential. After an agreement is attained, the resolution should be placed in writing and signed by participants.

42. D: Root cause analysis (RCA) is a retrospective attempt to determine the cause of an event, often a sentinel event such as an unexpected death, or a cluster of events. Root cause analysis involves interviews, observations, and review of medical records. Often, an extensive questionnaire is completed by the person doing the RCA, tracing essentially every step in hospitalization and care, including every treatment, every medication, and every contact. The focus of the RCA is on systems and processes rather than individuals.

43. B: If the state minimum wage is higher than the federal minimum wage under the Fair Labor Standards Act (FLSA), then the nurse executive must comply with the state minimum wage. The FLSA also sets standards for overtime pay for both full- and part-time workers. The FLSA applies to companies that engage in interstate commerce and whose businesses generate ≥$500,000 in annual dollar volume; however, hospitals and some other types of medical facilities and schools are covered by the Act regardless of the annual dollar volume.

44. D: A just organizational culture accepts that human error occurs and differentiates that from risky behavior and reckless behavior, also recognizing that errors are often the result of a system failure rather than an individual failure. In this case, the nurse made an inadvertent error and the correct response is to console the nurse. Risky behavior should result in coaching, such as sending the nurse for further training, while reckless behavior may require remedial or punitive action or even termination, depending on the extent of the reckless behavior, the cause, and the results to the patient.

45. C: While there may be value in all of these actions, probably the most effective is to schedule an open office hour for staff to drop in to discuss concerns. The reality is that the desire for access is often stronger than the actual need, so the nurse executive may find that much of the scheduled time can be used for other tasks, such as paperwork. Combining face-to-face access with email access is also effective because the nurse executive can look for recurring concerns and address those directly.

46. A: While all of these are elements of succession planning, the first step should be to describe the behaviors, skills, and leadership qualities necessary for the role. An

organization should have plans in place for both emergency and planned succession. Emergency succession most often identifies internal candidates with the skills and knowledge to fill a role, often on a temporary basis, while planned succession may focus on internal and/or external candidates, depending on organizational needs and future direction.

47. B: Because the goal of groupthink is consensus, the primary disadvantage is that it stifles dissent as organizational members feel pressure to conform, so important issues may not be adequately discussed. While groupthink is valuable in that it promotes harmony, allows focus on a single goal, and may help to implement new policies if supported by the majority, it often restricts creative solutions to problems and may result in resistance to major organizational changes.

48. C: The formula to determine the return on investment (ROI) is (Gain – Cost)/Cost: 113,000 – 100,000 = 13,000 divided by 100,000 = 0.13 or 13%. The ROI may be skewed if calculations do not include all costs, such as infrastructure costs, staffing, insurance, or maintenance costs. For example, if the new system required 10 additional hours of staff time per week at a cost of $80 per hour ($800 x 52 weeks), this would total an annual cost of $41,600, resulting in a loss of 28.6%.

49. C: Hospitals that receive Inpatient Prospective Payment System (IPPS) payments must complete 300 Hospital Consumer Assessment of Healthcare Providers and Systems (HCAHPS) surveys over the four calendar quarters of a year. The survey is given randomly to recently discharged (48 hours to 6 weeks) patients and contains 18 core questions about aspects of care and how satisfied patients were with the care they received. Surveys may be done by mail, telephone, mail plus telephone, or active-interactive voice recognition.

50. D: Nurses have the right to negotiate conditions of employment either as individuals or collectively (Right 7). Other rights include the right to:
1. Practice in such a way as to fulfill societal and patient obligations.
2. Practice in an environment in which they can maintain professional standards and work within their scope of practice.
3. Practice in an environment that supports and maintains ethical practice.
4. Advocate for patients/themselves without retribution.
5. Receive fair and appropriate compensation.
6. Work in a safe environment.

51. C: The nurse executive should first meet with the department administrator to gain valuable insight and information, to show respect for the person's position and experience, and to gain cooperation. However, the nurse executive cannot depend solely on the administrator's suggestions but should follow up with various types of needs assessments, including literature research, observation, interviews, surveys, and reviews of similar orientation programs. Expected outcomes should be identified in the process.

52. B: Studies have shown that the four things that motivate employees the most include:
- Autonomy: Allowing people to use their ideas.
- Salary: Providing adequate compensation for work done.
- Recognition: Appreciating the efforts that employees put forth.
- Respect: Listening to ideas.

A positive perception of leadership motivates people to produce and improve performance. In order to understand what motivates staff members, the leader must set aside preconceived ideas and listen carefully, discovering the strengths of the individuals and groups within the organization or facility and providing positive reinforcement and rewards.

53. C: Thirty percent of employees must sign the petition in order to file for an election. Upon receiving the petition and determining eligibility and jurisdiction, the NLRB meets with the employer to reach agreement over the time, place, type of ballot, ballot language, and eligibility criteria for the election to determine if the employees want to form or join a union. The election is usually held within 30 days once authorized, and the outcome of the election is determined by majority vote.

54. D: A Request for Information may be sent to vendors initially to facilitate comparison. The information should include all product details and specifications. Vendors should produce evidence of effective implementation of programs or equipment with similar organizations, provide a product history that includes the frequency of upgrades and the compatibility with previous software versions (if electronic), and provide product, maintenance, and service upgrades. The vendor should outline the type of support available and costs. Internet searches, networking, and conference attendance may also provide information.

55. D: Although it seems counterintuitive because of the cost of increasing the ratio of professional nurses to patients, according to the ANA, each additional RN actually results in an average of $60,000 savings over a year because of reduced medical costs associated with reduced rates of infection and other adverse events. Because patients receive better quality care, there is reduced risk of re-hospitalization and reduced malpractice claims. Additionally, staff satisfaction usually improves, resulting in less staff turnover.

56. A: A nurse executive who believes in Douglas McGregor's Theory X will probably favor an autocratic organizational culture. Theory X states that the average worker is unmotivated, dislikes work, is resistive to change, is unintelligent, and does not care about the organization. People work because they have to for money. Autocratic leaders make decisions independently, and strictly enforce rules, but staff members often feel left out of processes and may not be supportive. This type of leadership is most effective in crisis situations, but may have difficulty gaining commitment of staff.

57. D: The organizational chart shows the hierarchical system of the organization and relationships within that system. While the typical organizational chart is hierarchical, some organizations utilize a matrix format if there is more than one chain of command within an organization. Another format is horizontal, which is used in organizations in which all members have relatively equal input into decision making; however, this format is most commonly used within very small companies or individual units of a company.

58. D: There are two elements of crisis management that must be considered for internal and external disasters: reactive and preventive.
- Reactive elements include root cause analysis of observed problem, determination of long- and short-term effects, assignment of staff to deal with issues, and a search for improvement opportunities.

- Preventive elements include establishing control barriers, conducting direct observation and readiness activities, preparing contingency plans, and utilizing failure mode and effects analyses (FMEAs) for process design.

59. C: Under the patient-centered medical home model of care, patient care is coordinated through the primary care physician to establish a partnership between the patient/family and care givers. This physician coordinates all levels of patient care, including that provided by specialists. The primary care physician usually receives some additional compensation for this role in patient management. The goal is to ensure that the patient is viewed holistically and that problems are not overlooked or care fragmented in order to improve patient outcomes.

60. C: The Health Care Quality Improvement Act (HCQIA) of 1986 provides privacy protection for healthcare organizations and members engaged in peer review activities. While this act focused on peer review by physicians, the Omnibus Budget Reconciliation Act of 1991 expanded immunity to include non-physician peer evaluators as well:
- Healthcare personnel involved in formal peer review procedures, including performance improvement activities, are provided confidentiality and immunity in this process in order to further the quality of healthcare. Identifying information is excluded from reports and records. Certain conditions apply, and personnel are not exempted from suits/criminal action.

61. D: If a breach of privacy by a HIPAA-covered entity occurs, individuals must be notified as soon as possible and no later than 60 days. For fewer than 500 individuals, the U.S. Department of Health and Human Services must also be notified within 60 days of the end of the calendar year. If the breach involves 500 individuals or more, then the U.S. Department of Health and Human Services must be notified as soon as possible within 60 days of the breach and public notice made to broadcast media.

62. B: Offering or receiving a monetary reward of any kind, directly or indirectly, in return for a patient referral for Medicare or Medicaid reimbursable care is a violation of the Medicare and Medicaid Fraud and Abuse Law as outlined by the Anti-Kickback Statute (42 U.S.C. Section 1320a-7b(b)). Violations may result in prison terms of up to five years. Some payment practices are allowed under "safe harbor" regulations and are not considered violations. These can include rental space and equipment income, investment income, and recruitment payments.

63. C: Whistleblowers are protected under numerous federal (up to 20 different statutes) and state laws, which are sometimes contradictory and often confusing. Different laws apply to different occupations and subject matter. Depending upon the statute under which a person is acting as a whistleblower, different time limits for filing a complaint exist, so it's imperative that whistleblowers understand the laws that apply to them. In most cases, OSHA's Office of the Whistleblower Protection Program usually enforces statutes as delegated by the secretary of labor.

64. A: Team-based nursing usually involves teams of four to six members that include both professional nurses (such as RNs, and LVN/LPNs) and unlicensed assistive personnel (such as nurse's aides). The primary function of the team leader is to delegate tasks and provide supervision, as the team is responsible for the care of multiple patients. In some cases, team

leaders give direct care, such as administering medications and treatments, but in other cases, their role is primarily to coordinate care provided by other members of the team.

65. C: The nurse executive should first review acuity and census data, as the consistent need for overtime nursing hours suggests inadequate staffing for the needs of the unit. Assigning staff solely on the basis of bed count is often a poor strategy because one unit may have patients who are more ill and require more intensive care or may have many more admissions and discharges, which are both time consuming. Once armed with data, the nurse executive should meet with the Unit A administrator to find a resolution.

66. B: The resource-based relative value scale (RBRVS) system used by Medicare and HMOs is based on three factors: physician work, expense of practice, and expense of malpractice, with 52% based on work, 44% on practice, and 4% on malpractice expense. Physician's work includes consideration of such elements as time spent providing care, effort, education, and technical skill. A relative value is assigned according to geographic location, so that payments for the same CPT code may vary widely from one area to another.

67. A: A revenue cycle begins with admission of a patient and ends with final collection of unpaid bills. In a hospital, the most critical factor in the revenue cycle is the admission procedure. It is during admission that the patient's need for hospitalization should be verified and any necessary authorization from insurance companies obtained. Medicare, Medicaid, and insurance cards should be reviewed and coverage determined. If a patient has no insurance, then the responsible payor should be identified and a plan for payment discussed.

68. D: Model 4.
Model 1: Retrospective Acute Care Hospital Stay Only: Payment made for acute hospital care only.
Model 2: Retrospective Acute Care Hospital Stay plus Post-Acute Care: Payment for acute care and related services after discharge for 30, 60, or 90 days.
Model 3: Retrospective Post-Acute Care Only: Payment for post-acute services (including SNF, rehabilitation center, and home health care) beginning within 30 days of hospitalization and ending at 30, 60, or 90 days post-discharge.
Model 4: Acute Care Hospital Stay Only: Payment covers hospitalization, physician care and other practitioner's care. The hospital pays physicians and others out of the bundled payment.

69. B: The RN should report suspicions about the team leader to the next person in the chain of command, in this case the unit administrator, and should avoid confronting the team leader directly unless the person is impaired and actively putting patients in danger. The nurse administrator should receive the confidential report and act to determine if the team leader is impaired and/or diverting patient drugs. The nurse should not bypass the chain of command unless there is convincing evidence of complicity with illegal and/or unethical behavior by the next person in line.

70. B: Straight-line depreciation is calculated easily by taking the purchasing cost and subtracting the salvage value (the amount the equipment can be sold for when disposed of) and dividing that amount by the number of years of use ("useful life"). In this case:
$100,000 - $10,000 = $90,000 / 5 = $18,000.

With straight-line depreciation the depreciation is the same each year. Other methods of depreciation include declining balance, annuity depreciation, sum-of-year digits, units of time, group depreciation, and composite depreciation.

71. C: The Six Hats method is used to facilitate lateral thinking by encouraging six different ways of thinking and looking at a problem.
- White hat: Examining facts and figures and determining what information is needed and how to obtain it.
- Red hat: Focusing on feelings without explaining.
- Black hat: Making critical judgments and referring to rules and policies.
- Yellow hat: Viewing the situation positively and considering benefits.
- Green hat: Thinking creatively about different alternatives.
- Blue hat: Thinking about conclusions.

72. A: Zero-based: All cost centers are re-evaluated each budget period to determine if they should be funded or eliminated, partially or completely. Continuous/rolling: Periodic updates to the budget, including revenues, costs, volume, are done prior to the next budget cycle. Flexible: Estimates are made regarding anticipated changes in revenue and expenses and both fixed and variable costs are identified. Fixed/forecast: Revenue and expenses are forecast for the entire budget period and budget items are fixed.

73. B: SWOT analysis is used to evaluate internal and external factors that can affect work. Opposing factors are considered with (S) strengths and (W) weaknesses focused on internal factors and (O) opportunities and (T) threats on external factors. During SWOT analysis, a diagram is developed that outlines positive and negative opposing factors. Internal factors to consider include human resources, financial resources, processes, physical resources, and historical events. External factors to consider include the general economy, rules and laws, national/international events, demographics, sources of finances, and trends.

74. C: Category IC. Levels of evidence:
- Category IA: Well-supported by evidence from experimental, clinical, or epidemiologic studies and is strongly recommended for implementation.
- Category 1B: Supporting evidence from some studies, has a good theoretical basis, and strongly recommended for implementation.
- Category IC: Required by state or federal regulations or an industry standard.
- Category II: Supported by suggestive clinical or epidemiologic studies, has a theoretical basis, and is suggested for implementation.
- Category III: Supported by descriptive studies (such as comparisons, correlations, and case studies) and may be useful.
- Category IV: Obtained from expert opinion or authorities only.
- Unresolved: No recommendation because of a lack of consensus or evidence.

75. A: Pilot implementation is often used in large organizations or those with multiple locations to essentially "try out" the new system before it is further implemented. This is similar to phased rollout except that it is usually limited to one or a few units and extensive evaluation is usually completed during the pilot program, including interviews with users, to determine what faults exist and to assess end-user acceptance so that any alterations or modifications needed can be completed prior to further implementation.

76. B: Capital assets comprise durable assets (equipment, facilities) that are expected have an extended life and/or useful life span. When determining capital assets, each organization sets a capital threshold (in this case more than $600 and an expected life span (in this case more than 3 years), and only those items that fit both criteria are capital assets. The portable ultrasound meets the capital threshold and should have a life span of more than 3 years while the other items fail to meet both requirements.

77. D: Instituting a new streamlined discharge procedure for one unit fits the demands of intelligent risk taking because it's limited in scope so it's easy to determine the benefits (decreased demand for nursing time) versus the risks (inadequate preparation of patients for discharge). Purchasing facility-wide equipment without first testing runs the risk that the equipment might be unsuitable. Decreasing ICU nursing hours may result in increased costs because of deficient patient care. Announcing decreased benefits may result in widespread discontent and increased staff turnover.

78. B: Baby Boomers: Tend to be more self-centered but proactive and committed to ideas/causes but resistant to compromise with others. Generation X: Tend to be independent in thoughts and lifestyle, creative, and adaptive to change, but may overlook ethical concerns in the quest for achievement. Silent generation: Tend to be rule-oriented, cautious, and value trustworthiness and keeping one's word. They are practical and make decisions based on interest and opportunity. Millennial (Y) generation: Tend to believe they can be successful and are hardworking and confident in their abilities but may overlook the feelings and skills of others.

79. A: The digital dashboard is easy to access and integrates a variety of performance measures or key indicators into one display (usually with graphs or charts) to provide an overview of an organization. An organization-wide dashboard provides numerous benefits:
- Broad involvement of all departments.
- A consistent and easy to understand visual representation of data.
- Identification of negative findings or trends so that they can be corrected.
- Availability of detailed reports.
- Effective measurements that demonstrate the degree of efficiency.
- Assistance with making informed decisions.

80. C: A journal club meets on a regularly scheduled basis to read and evaluate articles in scientific and professional journals. Leadership elements include:
- Selecting appropriate articles to review: Articles should contain original research or metaanalysis and should contain a section regarding methods.
- Reviewing the articles completely, including evaluation of methods, materials, and outcomes and identifying the main points and conclusions of the article.
- Disseminating materials to all members at least a week prior to the meeting so they have time to study them.
- Leading the discussion, ensuring that all members participate, and determining the validity of the study and application to evidence-based practice.

81. B: The most important factor to consider when changing the skill mix to include more unlicensed assistive personnel is the experience of the professional nurses, because the nurses must assume more responsibility for delegating and supervising as well as evaluating patient needs. Nurses with a higher grade may have more education, but if they

lack experience in direct patient care or are new graduates, they may need mentoring and may not be ready for more responsibility.

82. A: Core criteria for credentialing and privileging include:
Performance ability: The person should have demonstrated ability to perform the duties to which the credentialing/privileging applies. Licensure: This must be current through the appropriate state board, such as the state board of nursing. Education: This includes training and experience appropriate for the credential and may include technical training, professional education, residencies, internships, fellowships, doctoral and post-doctoral programs, and board and clinical certifications. Competence: Evaluations and recommendations by peers regarding clinical competence and judgment provide information about how the person applies knowledge.

83. D: To facilitate quality improvement processes, the nurse executive should first secure support, resources, and approval from the governing board and key leaders. Other steps include:
- Build relationships among staff to facilitate change.
- Assess needs of the organizations, climate for change, and extent of support and resistance.
- Produce an internal action plan describing problems that need resolution, development needs, and process steps.
- Delineate resource needs, including staffing and training, with a detailed budget outlining all needs.
- Clarify roles and responsibilities organization-wide.
- Educate regarding the mission, vision, values, philosophy of quality management, techniques and tools, benefits, and accreditation and regulatory needs.

84. B: Coaching can include specific training, providing career information, and confronting issues of concern. Coaching should be done in a manner that increases learner confidence and ability to self-monitor rather than in a punitive or critical manner. An important element of coaching is using questioning to help the person recognize problem areas. Other elements include:
- Giving positive feedback, stressing what the person is doing right.
- Providing demonstrations and opportunities for question/answer periods.
- Providing regular progress reports so the person understands areas of concern.
- Assisting the person to establish personal goals for improvement.
- Providing resources to help the person master material.

85. C: External benchmarking involves analyzing data from outside an institution, such as monitoring national rates of hospital-acquired infection and comparing them to internal rates. In order for this data to be meaningful, the same definitions must be used as well as the same populations or effective risk stratification. Using national data can be informative, but each institution is different, and relying on external benchmarking to select indicators for infection control or other processes can be misleading. Additionally, benchmarking is a compilation of data that may vary considerably if analyzed individually, further compounded by anonymity that makes comparisons difficult.

86. A: Performance appraisal is used to confirm hiring, promote, train, or reward staff. It may be done on an annual basis and should be primarily based the person's job description,

which should include expectations and goals related to performance. The written appraisal should indicate compliance with performance expectations. The appraisal may include a rating scale, checklist, productivity studies, and narrative. The appraisal should be discussed with the individual so the person is able to respond. As part of the appraisal process, the individual should establish new goals, based on findings from performance improvement measures and related to strategic plans of the organization.

87. A: Shared governance implies shared decision making, but this can be realized in different ways. A common form of shared governance is for the administration to allow autonomous decision making by specific departments, teams, or groups within an organization regarding issues that apply to them or are within their area of expertise. For example, a unit team may have the authority to establish work schedules for that unit only, and members of a professional development team may be able to make decisions regarding professional development activities. In some cases, shared governance committees communicate with administration and can affect decision making but do not make the final decision.

88. D: Steps to developing evidence-based practice guidelines include:
1. Focus on the topic/methodology: Outline possible interventions/treatments for review, choosing patient populations and settings and determining significant outcomes.
2. Evidence review: Conduct literature review, critical analysis of studies, and summarizing of results.
3. Expert judgment: Allow, but this subjective evidence should be explicitly acknowledged.
4. Policy considerations: Include cost-effectiveness, access to care, insurance coverage, availability of qualified staff, and legal implications.
5. Policy: Complete a written policy with recommendations.
6. Review: Submit completed policy to peers for review and comments before instituting the policy.

89. C: "I understand you to say that you feel your working hours are excessive" paraphrases what the staff member has said without passing judgment. Active listening should focus on understanding the message and should avoid negative feedback or challenge but can include asking for clarification ("Could you explain that to me again?"). The listener should look directly at the speaker, nod and make brief comments ("uh huh," "yes," and "I see") and should avoid interrupting while the person is speaking.

90. C: Horizontal violence can include physical contact (such as hitting and shoving) but most often it involves verbal or non-verbal expressions of hostility and conflict, including defensive postures (folded arms) and gestures meant to show contempt (rolling the eyes). Horizontal violence is a form of workplace bullying and may include name-calling, sarcastic statements, blaming, ignoring other's concerns, making inappropriate jokes, and interfering with others rights as well as punishing others inappropriately. Horizontal violence may cause the victim to lose self-esteem, emotional control, and motivation.

91. A: Because burn patients are at high risk of infection, infection control is the most important factor to consider. The unit must be designed in such a way to prevent infection and cross-contamination while considering cost-effectiveness and workflow. Positive pressure must be maintained in the rooms as well as high levels of humidity (30 to 60%)

and high room temperatures (70 to 85%) to minimize fluid loss, so these technical concerns must be considered before staff preference. The design should be guided by an architect with expertise in designing burn units.

92. B: The best time for conflict resolution is when differences emerge but before open conflict and hardening of positions occur. Steps to conflict resolution include:
1. Allow both sides to present their side of conflict without bias, maintaining a focus on opinions rather than individuals.
2. Encourage cooperation through negotiation and compromise.
3. Maintain the focus, providing guidance to keep the discussions on track and avoid arguments.
4. Evaluate the need for renegotiation, formal resolution process, or third party.
5. Utilize humor and empathy to defuse escalating tensions.
6. Summarize the issues, outlining key arguments.
7. Avoid forcing resolution if possible

93. A: A hasty generalization is making an assumption about a group (women in OB) based on only one sample (Middle-Eastern patient). Overgeneralization is extending a conclusion beyond logical limits: "The nurse executive said this plan needs revision, so we should cancel it." Missing the point is suggesting the premise of an argument leads to a different conclusion from the one stated: "A higher professional staff mix leads to fewer infections, so we should fire all unlicensed assistive personnel." Appeal to ignorance is stating a belief is true if there is no clear evidence otherwise: "The patients with HIV in this unit were promiscuous."

94. C: Increasing the supplies budget for the department provides a solution to the problem but does not deal with the issue of cause. Critical thinking requires that problem solving be both solution-focused and cause-focused because dealing only with solutions often perpetuates the underlying problem. For example, if increased costs resulted from waste or stealing, the problem remains. Discussing the problem, conducting a study, and reviewing inventory procedures are all efforts to identify the cause of the increased costs and to determine if there is a legitimate need for an increased supplies budget.

95. D: With the PDSA cycle, Plan begins with extensive brainstorming to identify, analyze and define a problem. Fishbone diagrams or other mapping are used to identify problematic processes and list current process steps. Data is collected and analyzed and root cause analysis completed. Do generate solutions and one or more are implemented on a trial basis. Study (or Check) gathers and analyzes data to determine effectiveness of the trial solution. If ineffective, the participants return to Plan or choose a different solution and start the cycle again. Act identifies changes needed to fully implement an effective solution.

96. B: Patient/customer satisfaction is usually measured with surveys given to patients upon discharge or on completion of treatment. As patients become more knowledgeable and demand for accountability increases, patient satisfaction is being used as a guide for performance improvement although patient perceptions of clinical care do not always correlate with outcomes. The results of surveys can provide feedback that makes healthcare providers more aware of customer expectations. Currently, surveys are most often used to evaluate service elements of care rather than clinical elements.

97. B: Email notice is probably the most effective method for the nurse executive to employ to notify staff members of a meeting because most people have access to email at work, at home, or through a mobile device. The nurse can easily set up a mailing list, so notices can be sent out very quickly and at no cost. Mailed notices may be overlooked, and notices on bulletin boards are frequently ignored. Newsletters are often glanced at but not read in depth, so a notice there could be easily overlooked.

98. A: Ineffective communication is one of the primary causes of adverse events and malpractice claims. Studies show that the use of a standardized form or tool, such as SBAR, can markedly improve communication. While the sender should consider critical information and report verbally, the information should be organized and clear and time allowed for questions. SBAR tool:

(S) Situation: Overview of current situation and important issues.
(B) Background: Important history and issues leading to current situation.
(A) Assessment: Summary of important facts and condition.
(R) Recommendation: Actions needed.

Calls and direct hand-off should be documented, and orders reviewed by telephone read-back.

99. C: In reflective communication, the ability to perceive the mental processes of the self and others is referred to as mindsight. It involves the ability to be both empathetic and insightful. Reflective communication focuses on nurturing the other individual through positive responses and showing respect for the other's ideas and feelings. Reflective questions that can promote mindsight include "What are you thinking?" and "How do you feel about that?" Reflective communication requires openness to ideas, objective evaluation, and observation.

100. A: Feedback is a critical element of two-way communication, which comprises a sender, a message, a receiver, and feedback in a loop so that both the sender and the receiver receive feedback. One-way communication is a straight-line type of communication with a message sent and received without feedback. In an organization, formal communication (vertical) typically occurs from the top (administration) down (to staff) in a straight line and is typically delivered in a formal setting and/or in writing.

101. C: Passive-aggressive communication is exemplified by "Well, you're the boss, so I will do it your way" because the phrase suggests discontent without the person stating so directly. The passive-aggressive person often feels powerless and has difficulty being assertive but undermines or manipulates situations to try to influence outcomes. The passive-aggressive person often becomes very resentful of others, especially if the behavior is prompted by an environment that discourages open discussion or input and if the person feels his/her opinion is not valued.

102. C: The best communication method is probably a PowerPoint presentation. Issues include:

- Everyone in the room must be able to hear and see. In a large space, a projection screen must be used.
- Some projectors have low resolution and the lights need to be turned off /dimmed or windows covered, but this can be very distracting. A small portable light at a speaker podium or an alternate presentation can be used.

- PowerPoint or other presentations that include text must be of sufficient font size to be read from the back of the room.

103. C: Patient Self-Determination Act gives adults the right to refuse treatment, to direct treatment, and to prepare advance directives. Patients must be apprised of their rights on admission to a Medicare or Medicaid provider, such as a hospital. Older Americans Act provides improved access to services for older adults and Native Americans, including community services, such as transportation and meals. Americans with Disabilities Act provides the disabled, including those with mental impairment, access to employment and the community. Emergency Medical Treatment and Active Labor Act (EMTALA) is designed to prevent patient "dumping" from emergency departments.

104. C: Progressive nursing care is a model of care in which patients are placed in units according to their needs for care rather than their diagnosis. In a typical model, levels of care include ICU for seriously ill patients, self-care for those who are still convalescing or are being evaluated, intermediate care for those who don't fit the other models (more than half of patients), and outpatient short stay for those who require a stay of less than 24 hours.

105. B: Clinical/critical pathways are specific multi-disciplinary care plans that outline interventions and outcomes of diseases, conditions, and procedures. Clinical pathways are based on data and literature and best practices. The expected outcomes are delineated as well as the sequence of interventions and the timeline needed to achieve the outcomes. There are many different types of forms that appear similar to flow sheets but are more complex and require more documentation. Any variance from the pathway or expected outcomes must be documented. Clinical pathways are increasingly used to comply with insurance limitations to ensure cost-effective timely treatment.

106. D: A patient who is able to drive somewhere routinely and take classes is probably not going to be considered homebound. Criteria for homebound status include recommendation to not leave home, the need for help when leaving home (wheelchair, walker, assistance), and/or a taxing effort required to leave home. Patients are allowed to leave home to receive medical treatments and may have short infrequent absences from home for other purposes, such as to attend religious services. Adult day care does not preclude a patient from being classified as homebound.

107. B: A targeted approach focuses on the needs of one or a group of similar patients. In this case, a series of classes is set up specifically to address the needs of COPD patients in order to reduce re-hospitalization. With a targeted approach, the facilitator should establish group goals (reduce re-hospitalization by 75%) as well as individual goals (demonstrate purse-lipped and diaphragmatic breathing). While posters, public education via television, and booklets on discharge are also useful, they are likely to have less impact than classes.

108. B: Because most core measures are related to adult health issues, freestanding children's hospitals must collect data on only one core measure (Children's Asthma Care) and nine non-core measures. General and critical care hospitals are required to collect data on four core measures or a combination of core and non-core measures. Measure sets include Acute Myocardial Infarction, Heart Failure, Pneumonia, Perinatal Care, Hospital-Based Inpatient Psychiatric Services, Surgical Care Improvement Project, Hospital Outcome Measures, Venous Thromboembolism, Stroke, Emergency Department, Tobacco Treatment, Immunization, and Substance Abuse.

109. D: Sentinel events are deaths or serious physical injuries that are unexpected. Sentinel events could be related to many things, including surgery on the wrong body part, in-hospital suicide, or infection. Infections are considered sentinel events if the death or injury would not have occurred without the infection. Each case must be dealt with individually, and, if defined as sentinel, a root cause analysis that defines the problem through gathering evidence to identify what contributed to the problem must be done, followed by an action plan that identifies all the different elements that contributed to the problem.

110. D: A healthy work environment provides nurturing of the staff in order to achieve good patient outcomes and excellence in clinical care. A healthy work environment includes receiving meaningful recognition, which helps people to feel valued. Other essential elements include a true effort at collaboration and effective decision making. In order for these elements to be successful, skilled communication is essential. Authentic leadership responds appropriately to needs and must allow for appropriate and adequate staffing.

111. C: The Joint Commission has established leadership standards that apply to healthcare organizations and help to establish management's lines of authority and accountability. Under these standards, leadership comprises the governing body, the chief executive officer and senior managers, department leaders, leaders (both elected and appointed) of staff or departments, and the nurse executive and other nurse leaders. The governing body is ultimately responsible for all patient care rendered by all types of practitioners (physicians, nurses, laboratory staff, support staff) within and under the jurisdiction of the organization.

112. D: Back-end e-health exchange of data does not directly involve the patient as a participant, such as occurs when a physician requests medical records or laboratory reports electronically even though this is for the benefit of the patient. Front-end e-health exchange does involve the patient and may include the patient emailing a physician directly or sending a photo of a rash or injury in order to obtain medical advice. This type of data exchange can save time and costs although privacy remains a major concern.

113. C: While mentoring may entail a long-term relationship and coaching and training are usually focused on specific skills, precepting is usually a time-limited arrangement related to a term of study, such as a semester, orientation period, or a clinical rotation. The preceptor must be able to provide adequate clinical supervision and guidance to the student on a daily basis. This may require coordinating schedules and planning carefully to ensure all responsibilities can be met. The preceptor may engage in shared care as well as direct supervision in order to improve the student's skills.

114. A: Emotional intelligence can be described by different models, but an early model is that of Salovoy and Mayer, who described four different types of abilities associated with emotional intelligence:
- Ability to perceive emotions: To look at a person's facial expression and to understand and perceive that person's emotions.
- Ability to use emotions: To use emotions and changing moods to improve problem solving and thinking processes.
- Ability to understand emotions: To comprehend and be sensitive to the subtleties of emotion.
- Ability to manage emotions: To control emotions of the self and others.

- 46 -

115. A: Nursing is a high-stress profession, and almost all nurses benefit from informal peer support from others in the profession through discussion and networking. Formal peer support groups are becoming more common as the profession recognizes that nurses must often cope with psychologically traumatic experiences as part of their profession as well as in their personal lives. Formal peer support groups may comprise members from various levels of the organization, but when possible the members should be chosen by staff rather than assigned.

116. D: The most important element of the pro forma business plan is the business activity, which describes the type of business and the product or service the business will produce as well as future plans. The rest of the plan should relate directly to the business activity. Business aims should outline broad goals while the business objectives should contain more specific targets. Business market should contain an explanation of the market research that has been conducted and the potential market for the product or services.

117. B: The premise of servant leadership is that the leader is not meant to simply exercise power and make decisions but to serve all those within the organization and/or community. Leadership is considered an altruistic endeavor. Thus, essential qualities of a servant leader include the ability to listen effectively to the input of others and to exercise empathy, always putting the organizational needs and greater good above personal needs. The leader needs to have a good sense of self-awareness and the ability to persuade and influence others.

118. A: Corporate compliance means that controls are in place in an organization to prevent violations of rules, laws, and regulations, usually through active risk management and application of ethical standards. Organizations must have procedures in place to mitigate illegal conduct, with high-level personnel tasked with assessing and assuring compliance, preventing access of discretionary authority to those who are at risk for illegal conduct. Staff must be aware of standards and procedures, as well as steps taken to achieve compliance and enforcement of policies and to act if misconduct occurs.

119. A: Knowledge management refers to methods to share and manage information. Push strategies involve developing strategies, such as building a database of information, to actively control and manage the information so that it can be literally "pushed" to various database users. Push strategies are generally codified. Pull, on the other hand, involves taking information directly from a source, such as having an expert providing guidance or information to those individuals or groups who need it. Pull strategies are generally personified.

120. B: Leadership, both on the part of the nurse executive and other nurse administrators and physicians, is the most critical element in creating a culture of staff accountability. Leaders must communicate values and a shared vision that emphasizes quality of care and quality in all aspects of the organization with customer service as a priority. The organization must continually assess and measure performance while clarifying roles and expectations and ensuring there is infrastructure support.

121. A: While all of these have a role, the most important is to maintain and improve professional skills. Each state sets requirements for continuing education for licensure renewal and some certification agencies also require the nurse to take a specific number of hours of continuing education as well. In addition, specific courses may be required by employers for job-related purposes. ANCC uses six categories of professional development,

and candidates must complete hours in at least two categories: CE hours, academic credits, presentations, research or publications, precepting, or professional service.

122. D: The nurse executive should assume that no assumption about the person can be made without further information and observation. Making eye contact provides a connection and shows caring and involvement in the communication. Avoiding contact may indicate someone is not telling the truth or is uncomfortable, fearful, ashamed, or hiding something. However, in some cultures (Asian, Native American, African American), eyes are averted as a sign of respect. Without knowing the person and the person's background and usual behavior, one should not make assumptions based only on failure to make eye contact.

123. B: To qualify for treatment in an inpatient rehabilitation facility (IRF) a patient must meet medical necessity requirements, which include the potential to benefit from therapy and the need for multiple therapies (at least one must be physical therapy or occupational therapy) with at least 3 hours of daily rehabilitation therapy 5 days a week or 15 hours in a consecutive 7-day period (if well-documented). Note that no rounding up of minutes in reporting therapy time is permitted. Therapy disciplines can include physical therapy, occupational therapy, speech/language pathology, or prosthetics/orthotics.

124. A: Negotiating of any kind requires willingness to compromise, so going to negotiations with an intransigent outcome in mind usually results in prolonged conflict. The nurse executive should know at the beginning of negotiations what the desired outcome (best case) is as well as the minimum acceptable outcome (worst case) because the settlement area lies between those two extremes. The nurse executive should listen completely to the other side, showing respect, while still being assertive but willing to compromise. For win-win negotiation, both sides must achieve at least part of their goal outcome.

125. C: When complaints arise regarding interpersonal relations among staff, the best initial action is to address those concerns with the person in a one-on-one conversation. The nurse executive should outline the complaints in a non-punitive manner while at the same time reinforcing organizational policies regarding ethical treatment of staff. A good approach is to ask, "What can I do to help you?" In many cases, behavior changes result from stresses that may not be job related, such as financial concerns or family illness.

126. A: An advisory committee does not establish new procedures or make policies, so the primary role of a patient/family advisory council is to address the needs of patients/families and provide valuable feedback about the experience of being a patient or family member. While some feedback may include deficiencies in care, this is not the primary focus. The advisory committee can bring a fresh perspective and new ideas to influence policies and procedures.

127. C: "That's an interesting idea, but here are the problems…." shows respect for the other person but states clearly the issues. Statements that devalue others, such as "That's a ridiculous idea" and "You should know that won't work" are aggressive and often increase resistance or result in resentment. Passively agreeing to try an unworkable solution is a sign of weakness and lack of confidence. Also, a passive communication style can result in wasted time, as the person may be afraid to make decisions.

128. D: CQMs provide lists of measures to be assessed as well as expectations related to care. The CQM Population/Public Health focuses on screening and preventive measures, such as

"weight assessment and counseling for nutrition and physical activity for children and adolescents." For example, this measure assesses in percentages the patients (age 3 to 17) who saw a physician and had evidence in the electronic health record of height, weight, and BMI (percentile) and those who received counseling for nutrition and counseling for physical activity.

129. B: The goal of service recovery is to satisfy the customer/client and retain that person's good will and loyalty when a mistake has occurred. The first step when the mistake is pointed out is to apologize immediately, without trying to deny the mistake or make excuses. The next step is to do what is necessary to rectify the problem and, when appropriate, to offer some type of compensation or service that will have value to the customer/client.

130. D: One of the most effective ways to network is to become involved in national organizations and to participate in conferences through attendance and conference presentations. The executive nurse should make an effort to maintain periodic contact with those in an informal network by telephone, mail, or email, or social networking sites, such as LinkedIn and Facebook, but the nurse must use care not to violate confidentiality and privacy and should avoid posting negative statements. Personal and professional sites should be kept separate and private sites password protected.

131. A: The nurse executive can use the STAR method to communicate program improvement and increase visibility in a succinct organized manner. While this method is often used as an interview technique, it can be used to communicate progress (or failures) for most situations. The steps to the STAR Method include:
- Situation: Problem recognition, circumstances.
- Task: Needed outcomes and specific required actions.
- Action: Specific details about what was actually done to meet the tasks.
- Results: Success or failures, including measurements.

132. D: The most significant barrier to development of a culture of transparency to improve patient safety is fear of punitive action or retribution. A culture of transparency means that staff members must be alert to at-risk situations and errors and be willing to identify and report both, whether resulting from their own actions, actions of others, or systemic problems. However, if administration reacts by taking punitive action, many staff members, fearing for their jobs or the jobs of others, are reluctant to report concerns. Thus, an important aspect of a culture of transparency may be instituting a just culture.

133. D: The balanced scorecard (Kaplan and Norton) is based on the strategic plan and provides performance measures in relation to the mission and vision statement and goals and objectives. A balanced scorecard includes not only the traditional financial information but also includes data about customers, internal processes, and education/learning. Each organization can select measures that help to determine if the organization is on track to meeting its goals. If the scorecard is adequately balanced, it will reflect both the needs and priorities of the organization itself and also those of the community and customers.

134. A: Four types of strategic planning data:
- Aggregate: Pharmacy transactions, required reports, demographic information, financial information, hazard and safety practices, and most things not included in the clinical record.

- 49 -

- Medical/clinical: Patient-specific including information regarding diagnosis, treatment, laboratory findings, consultations, care plans, physician orders, medical records, and information related to informed consent and advance directives.
- Knowledge-based: Methods to ensure that staff is provided training, support, research, library services or other access to information, and good practice guidelines.
- Comparisons: This data may relate to internal comparisons or external comparisons to benchmarks or best-practice guidelines.

135. A: Under the Affordable Care Act Patient's Bill of Rights, insurance companies may not retroactively cancel the policy of a patient who becomes ill in order to avoid paying for care. Health plans must provide coverage for all children who apply, regardless of pre-existing conditions. Lifetime limits for compensation have been eliminated and phased elimination of annual limits is occurring although some plans with annual limits are grandfathered in. Currently, balanced billing may still occur if people seek care outside of the provider network.

136. C: Identification of variances from baseline data first requires baseline data that is representative for the target population. This involves an initial period of surveillance and review. Baseline data can be established for various periods of time, but a one-month period is commonly used. Threshold rates should also be established. Once the baseline is established, new data is analyzed to determine if there are variances (changes), usually increases, although decreases may be identified if data is collected for the purpose of charting improvements.

137. B: ANA Code of Ethics:
1. Treat all patients with respect and consideration.
2. Retain primary commitment to the patient regardless of conflicts.
3. Promote and advocate for the patient's health, safety, and rights, maintaining privacy, confidentiality, and protecting them from questionable practices or care.
4. Remain responsible for own care practices and determine appropriate delegation of care.
5. Retain respect for self and one's own integrity and competence.
6. Ensure the healthcare environment is conducive to providing good health care, consistent with professional and ethical values.
7. Participate in education and knowledge development.
8. Collaborate with others.
9. Articulate values and promote and maintain the integrity of the profession.

138. D: The primary goal of a bioethics committee is to determine the most morally correct action using the set of circumstances given. If the patients/parents and the staff are in agreement when it comes to values and decision making, then no ethical dilemma exists; however, when there is a difference in value beliefs between the patients/parents and the staff, there is a bioethical dilemma that must be resolved. Sometimes, discussion and explanation can resolve differences, but at times the institution's bioethics committee must be brought in to resolve the conflict.

139. B: Reasons for forming performance improvement teams include:
- To improve outcomes through common purpose.
- To utilize staff expertise and various perspectives.

- To facilitate participative management style.
- To improve acceptance of processes that impact work practice.
- To manage complexity, where many participants are involved in outcomes.
- To increase organization-wide acceptance.
- To combat resistance.

Performance improvement activities almost always involve a team or teams of staff because of the complexity of healthcare organizations. Rarely is one department solely responsible for outcomes, except in very specialized work.

140. C: Triggers are mechanisms or signals within data that indicate when further analysis (such as case review or root cause analysis) or prioritizing needs to be done, and these triggers should be selected for each measure of performance. External triggers include benchmarks, feedback from staff and internal and external customers, strategic planning initiatives, planning guidelines, and research. Internal triggers include sentinel events, performance rate, rate change, difference between groups, specified upper and lower control limits about a mean, and control limits.

141. B: "You don't need to worry about that. You will receive medications to control the adverse effects" is not responsive to the patient's question and does not provide informed consent. The American Medical Association has established guidelines for informed consent:
- Explanation of diagnosis.
- Nature and reason for treatment or procedure.
- Risks and benefits.
- Alternative options (regardless of cost or insurance coverage).
- Risks and benefits of alternative options.
- Risks and benefits of not having a treatment or procedure.

Providing informed consent is a requirement of all states.

142. C: Specific data about individual patients or healthcare workers are often protected by laws regarding privacy, so information about individuals cannot be disseminated unless anonymity can be assured. Reports to individual physicians about their own effectiveness rates should be provided confidentially and comparison rates done without identifying physicians. Reports with identifying information removed when necessary are usually presented to the administration and teams, but reports should also be presented to staff in areas of survey so that staff and physicians are aware of the study results and can evaluate the effectiveness of procedures or institute preventive methods.

143. D: The four Ds of appreciative inquiry are (1) discover, (2) dream, (3) design, and (4) destiny/ deliver. The primary focus of appreciative inquiry is on the positive aspects of an organization, so the purpose of inquiry is not to assess that which is wrong or to fix problems but to assess that which is successful so that these aspects can be emphasized and emulated, thereby eliminating problems. Inquiry is often conducted through interviews with staff members, either individually or in groups.

144. A: While all of these trends have impacted the delivery of healthcare, technological advances have had a profound effect. Developments include telehealth, electronic health records, automated medication dispensing carts, robotic surgery, and electronic monitoring. Record storage and access to records have been transformed but with this comes increasing

concerns about privacy and dissemination of information. The Internet provides healthcare providers and consumers immediate information, both accurate and inaccurate. Nursing education must change to meet this trend, and nurses require almost continuous ongoing training for new equipment and processes.

145. B: Contingency theory states that there is no one best method of leadership but that a leader's skill must match the needs of the situation, which is contingent on a number of different factors, so what works in one organization may not work in another. Some common contingency factors include the organization size, resources, technology, adaptation to the environment, operations activities, motivating forces, staff education, and managerial assumptions. Contingency theory states that the organization must be designed in such a manner as to fit into the environment, and management should utilize the best approach to achieve tasks.

146. B: The FDA maintains and regulates procedures and recall regarding contaminated equipment and supplies a website entitled MedWatch to provide safety information for drugs and medical equipment. MedWatch provides electronic listing service to medical professionals and facilities for the following:
- Medical product safety alerts.
- Information about drugs and devices.
- Summary of safety alerts with links to detailed information.

Facilities must file semiannual reports on January 1 and July 1 and must maintain records for two years and develop written procedures for identification, evaluation, and submission of medical device reports (MDR). MedWatch provides reporting forms for voluntary and mandatory reports.

147. D: The case manager is responsible for screening patients from the time of admission (or before admission in some cases) and assisting with planning for discharge. Within an acute, sub-acute, or skilled nursing facility, the case manager may chair the interdisciplinary team to ensure that the needs of the patient are communicated and that all members of the team are focused on similar goals. The case manager needs to consider the social support services (home health care, transportation, Meals-on-Wheels) that are needed for the person to remain as independent as possible and to function safely after discharge.

148. D: While all of these are important, self-awareness is essential to understanding potential biases because people tend to believe that their own belief system is superior to others. Studies indicate that those who are diverse, that is ethnic, cultural, or lifestyle minorities, are often treated differently by healthcare providers in the sense that they may receive less than optimal care. The nurse executive must also ask staff to assess their own attitudes and encourage open discussions about differences to help people to gain self-awareness and determine if their ideas are stereotypical and/or based on lack of knowledge.

149. D: Steps to critical reading for research:
1. Consider the source. Popular press has little validity compared to a juried journal.
2. Review the author's credentials to determine if the person is an expert in the field of study.
3. Determine thesis, or central claim of the research.
4. Examine the organization of the article, whether it is based on a particular theory, and the type of methodology used.

5. Review the evidence to determine how it supports the main points. Look for statistical evidence and sample size.
6. Evaluate the overall article to determine credibility and usefulness.

150. C: The grant applicant should have a clear idea of the type of research project and begin to collect preliminary data and identify those who will supervise or participate in the project before applying. Steps include:

- Review all directions and written material and follow the directions exactly.
- Begin application process early to allow time for revisions.
- Establish a clear timeline.
- Provide detailed budget information, including support staff (such as office workers) and supplies, outlining exactly the budget for each year of the project.
- Provide a comprehensive literature review.
- Write clearly and proofread to ensure there are no grammatical errors.

Practice Test #2

Practice Questions

1. How many community members who are unaffiliated with the organization must be included in an Institutional Review Board to meet FDA requirements?
    a. 1.   *minimal of 5 members total*
    b. 2.   *including a community member.*
    c. 3.
    d. 4.

2. The first step in strategic planning is:
    a. developing a revised mission and vision statement that identifies core values.
    b. establishing specific goals and objectives.
    c. analyzing internal services and functions
    d. collecting data and doing an external analysis of customer needs.

3. The Joint Commission's Environment of Care requires management plans for which functional areas?
    a. Safety, security, hazardous materials and waste, fire safety, medical equipment, and utilities.
    b. Pharmacy, medical equipment, ventilation, and hazardous materials and waste.
    c. Infection control, fire safety, discharge planning, security, and technology.
    d. Infection control, safety, security, ventilation, pharmacy, and medical equipment.

4. Under the Transtheoretical Model stages of change, the stage during which the person intends to change at some point and is aware of costs and benefits of change is called:
    a. Precontemplation.
    b. Contemplation.
    c. Preparation.
    d. Action.

5. The nurse manager of the emergency department routinely makes homeless or indigent patients wait for care until other patients have been seen. What provision of the American Nurse Association Nursing Code of Ethics does this specifically violate?
    a. The nurse is responsible for his/her own care practices and determines appropriate delegation of care.
    b. The nurse's primary commitment is to the patient regardless of conflicts that may arise.
    c. The nurse must retain respect for self and his/her own integrity and competence.
    d. The nurse treats all patients with respect and consideration, regardless of social circumstances or health condition.

- 54 -

6. Which of the following terms refers specifically to the process by which a person is granted authority to practice in an organization?
    a. Licensing
    b. Privileging
    c. Credentialing
    d. Certifying

7. In Juran's 4-step quality improvement process (QIP), which of the following is done as part of the *remediating* step?
    a. Prioritizing problems and identifying a team.
    b. Analyzing problems and formulating theories.
    c. Considering various alternative solutions.
    d. Evaluating performance and monitoring control system.

8. The initial enrollment period for Medicare part D for a 45-year old disabled patient who is newly eligible for Medicare is:
    a. 3 months prior to Medicare eligibility and 4 months after.
    b. Months 21 through 27 after receiving Social Security or Railroad Retirement Board (RRB) benefits.
    c. April 1 to June 30.
    d. 3 months prior to Medicare eligibility and 7 months after.

9. Under the CMS Inpatient Rehabilitation Facility Prospective Payment System (IFR PPS), an impairment group is grouped according to:
    a. The same impairment category.
    b. Similar age, motor functioning, and cognitive ability.
    c. The number of comorbidities.
    d. The type of comorbidity.

10. Nurses, at the end of each shift, are required to give each of their patients a score based on their needs for care. This is commonly a component of which type of staffing model?
    a. Skill mix
    b. Primary care
    c. Team nursing
    d. Acuity-based

11. With Medicare, the benefit period ends:
    a. 60 days after discharge from an inpatient facility.
    b. 30 days after discharge from an inpatient facility.
    c. at the time of discharge from an inpatient facility.
    d. 150 days after discharge from an inpatient facility.

12. The type of healthcare insurance that pays in the form of predetermined payments for loss or damages rather than for healthcare services is called:
    a. liability insurance.
    b. no-fault auto insurance.
    c. indemnity insurance.
    d. accident and health insurance.

13. The purpose of stop-loss insurance is to:
   a. protect the insurance company against excessive payments.
   b. defer medical expenses until a time when funds become available.
   c. replace a part of insurance coverage and may exclude certain treatments.
   d. limit the types of services covered.

14. When an insurance plan negotiates a specific fee for a procedure (including all charges) and pays one bill, this is referred to as:
   a. unbundling.
   b. bundling.
   c. fee-for-service.
   d. discounted fee-for-service.

15. The nurse executive proposes conducting a market survey to determine the need for a new clinic, the types of services to be offered, and the best location for the clinic. Which healthcare supply system is the nurse executive utilizing?
   a. Market-driven
   b. Provider-driven
   c. Supply-driven
   d. Profit-driven

16. Under a healthcare management program for diabetics, a targeted approach to reducing diabetic complications includes:
   a. hanging posters in physician's office.
   b. creating television commercials.
   c. participating in a community health fair.
   d. providing nutritional counseling.

17. The first step in developing a healthcare management program is to:
   a. identify resources.
   b. develop strategies.
   c. define the population.
   d. determine outcomes measurement.

18. In a subacute facility, a stroke patient that requires 20 days of care and rehabilitation and/or nursing services for four hours a day is categorized as:
   a. chronic subacute.
   b. general subacute.
   c. transitional subacute.
   d. long-term transitional subacute.

19. When conducting a survey for program evaluation, the easiest questions to quantify are:
   a. descriptive informational questions (who, what, when, were, how, how much, why).
   b. yes-no questions.
   c. multiple choice questions.
   d. based on a rating scale.

20. The primary core criteria for credentialing and privileging are:
    a. licensure, education, competence, and performance ability.
    b. licensure, education, quality of care, and clinical knowledge.
    c. licensure, education, communication skills, and professionalism.
    d. licensure, education, clinical knowledge, and systems knowledge.

21. Denial or noncertification of services may result from:
    a. extended hospitalization because of postoperative myocardial infarction.
    b. extended hospitalization because PT is not available on the weekends.
    c. change in policy after services rendered.
    d. client's death.

22. The Older American's Act provides funding and support for:
    a. hospital services.
    b. pharmacy assistance programs.
    c. home and community services.
    d. financial assistance to older adults.

23. Upon discharge from a hospital, the most appropriate placement for a client who has slight dementia and requires a daily simple dry dressing change but is medically stable and ambulates independently with a cane is:
    a. a subacute/rehabilitation facility.
    b. a skilled nursing facility.
    c. an intermediate care facility.
    d. an assisted living/custodial care facility.

24. An example of unskilled care is:
    a. administering sliding scale insulin.
    b. educating a client about a low sodium diet.
    c. instructing in the use of assistive devices.
    d. taking and reporting routine vital signs.

25. An action plan has been formulated that clearly outlines the expected outcomes, the steps in the plan, designated responsibilities, anticipated timeline, and the types of measurements to be used for monitoring and evaluating. What is the next step?
    a. Conduct pilot testing.
    b. Train all staff and institute organization-wide changes at one time.
    c. Begin to implement the action plan on a trial basis.
    d. Establish a timeline for full implementation.

26. When a facility is converting to the interoperable electronic healthcare delivery system, the most important aspect to consider is:
    a. equipment choice.
    b. time needed for conversion.
    c. staff training.
    d. staff preference.

27. The level of care that provides people with moderate assistance in activities of daily living and periodic nursing supervision for some activities is called:
    a. custodial care.
    b. intermediate care.
    c. skilled nursing.
    d. acute care.

28. Two staff nurses disagree about the best way to carry out their duties, resulting in ongoing conflict and refusal to work together. The first step in resolving this conflict is to:
    a. allow both individuals to present their side of the conflict without bias.
    b. encourage them to reach a compromise.
    c. tell them they are violating professional standards of conduct.
    d. make a decision about the matter.

29. The primary criterion for referral to a hospice program is
    a. severe intractable pain.
    b. a life-threatening disease.
    c. the probability that death will occur within 6 months.
    d. the presence of a DNR order.

30. There is only one bed available in a skilled nursing facility, but there are two patients who are in need of care. The nurse recommends that one patient be transferred to another facility. The decision regarding which patient to transfer should be based on which ethical principle?
    a. Nonmaleficence
    b. Beneficence.
    c. Justice.
    d. Autonomy.

31. Which of the following laws require that communities provide transportation services for the disabled, including accommodations for wheelchairs?
    a. Emergency Medical Treatment and Active Labor Act (EMTALA).
    b. Older Americans Act (OAA).
    c. Omnibus Budget Reconciliation Act (OBRA).
    d. Americans with Disabilities Act (ADA).

32. Which of the following violates the American Medical Association's guidelines for informed consent?
    a. Description of risks and benefits of treatment.
    b. Presentation of only the 3 most cost-effective treatment options.
    c. Review of the nature of treatment and purpose.
    d. Comparison of success rates for similar treatment at different facilities.

33. Which of the following best describes a case mix group as defined by the Health Insurance Prospective Payment System (HIPPS)?
    a. A classification system based on utilization of resources.
    b. A data set containing elements to review for a comprehensive assessment of patient function.
    c. A classification system based on clinical characteristics of patients.
    d. A data set used by home health agencies to measure outcomes and risk factors.

- 58 -

34. The primary purpose of sending a request for information (RFI) to multiple vendors is to:
   a. aid in the elimination and selection process.
   b. meet regulatory requirements.
   c. eliminate the need for a request for quote (RFQ).
   d. complete a cost-utility analysis.

35. The first step to knowledge discovery in a database (KDD) is:
   a. data mining.
   b. data selection.
   c. pre-processing data.
   d. transforming data.

36. According to the Health Information Technology for Economic and Clinical Health Act (HITECH) security provisions, a breach in security of personal health information requires notification of:
   a. administration.
   b. the physician.
   c. the US Department of Health and Human Services (HHS).
   d. the individuals impacted and US Department of Health and Human Services (HHS).

37. Which of the following is an example of intelligent risk taking when a nurse executive is faced with the need to cut costs?
   a. Switching to an acuity-based nursing care model to reduce overtime costs.
   b. Reducing nursing staff across the board in all departments.
   c. Reducing support staff by 50%.
   d. Hiring all part-time staff to avoid paying benefits.

38. The communication theory that describes communication as an exchange system in which people attempt to negotiate a return on their "investment" in much the same way that people engage in commerce is:
   a. Social Penetration Theory (Altman and Taylor).
   b. Communication Accommodation Theory (Giles).
   c. Spiral of Science Theory (Noelle-Neuman).
   d. Social Exchange Theory (Homans, Thibaut, and Kelley).

39. Which of the following serves as the guide for tracer methodology?
   a. Patient surveys
   b. Patient medical records
   c. Staff surveys
   d. Accreditation reports

40. The primary purpose of knowledge management is to:
   a. increase organizational effectiveness.
   b. widely disseminate information.
   c. provide safeguards to prevent unauthorized access to information.
   d. codify and transmit data.

41. The Leapfrog Safe Practices score is used as a basis for:
   a. Promoting evidence-based practice through the funding of 14 Evidence-based Practice Centers (EPCs).
   b. Providing collaborative training within the network related to safe clinical practice.
   c. Providing fellowships to help professionals gain experience and expertise in health-related fields.
   d. Assessing progress a healthcare organization is making on 30 safe practices.

42. The employee assistance program's critical incident stress management (CISM) plan is initiated after a severe explosion and fire brings dozens of critically injured patients to the hospital. When should the defusing sessions begin?
   a. As soon as possible during or after the event
   b. Two to three days after the event
   c. One week after the event
   d. Within 2 weeks after the event

43. A nurse executive's span of control refers to:
   a. the type of governance.
   b. the number of patients.
   c. the number of subordinate staff who report to her.
   d. the number of departments she manages.

44. The National Quality Forum's safe practices, specifically regarding medication management, includes:
   a. the need to document care properly.
   b. implementing a computerized prescriber order entry (CPOE) system.
   c. informing patients of medication side effects and risks.
   d. providing discharge planning.

45. In a database, the type of data that is usually used to represent a count of something is:
   a. categorical.
   b. quantitative.
   c. discrete.
   d. continuous.

46. When brainstorming as part of action planning, which of the following is the first step?
   a. Establish the purpose of and the time frame to brainstorm.
   b. List every suggested idea.
   c. Discuss items and clarify issues.
   d. Decide on a structured or unstructured approach.

47. Which of the following legal procedures authorizes disclosure of patient personal health information?
   a. Subpoena
   b. Subpoena duces tecum
   c. Warrant
   d. Court order

- 60 -

48. The nurse executive would find Workers' Compensation data most useful when researching which of the following?
   a. Tracking occupational illness.
   b. Determining safety measures.
   c. Estimating frequency of particular occupational injuries.
   d. Reducing costs of work-related injuries.

49. The four necessary elements of all negligence claims are:
   a. Duty to care, harm, liability, and residual damages.
   b. Onset, duration, cause, and injury.
   c. Victim, perpetrator, injury, and residual damages.
   d. Duty of care, breach of duty, damages, and causation.

50. According to von Bertalanffy's Systems Theory, which of the following is an example of throughput?
   a. Raw materials
   b. Planning processes
   c. Rules
   d. Accreditation reports

51. A sentinel event occurs when an 80-year-old post-operative patient develops a *Clostridium difficile* infection and dies as a result of the infection. The first step in preventing further cases is to:
   a. conduct a root cause analysis.
   b. develop an action plan.
   c. close the unit for extensive cleaning.
   d. educate staff about infection control measures.

52. When conducting a stakeholder analysis as part of long-term planning, the initial step is to:
   a. evaluate stakeholders.
   b. map stakeholder relationships.
   c. identify important stakeholders.
   d. classify stakeholders as either primary or secondary.

53. The Hospital Compare Internet site provided by Medicare allows for the comparison of how many different hospitals at one time?
   a. 2
   b. 3
   c. 5
   d. 10

54. When reviewing data provided by the CMS Hospital Quality Initiative, the nurse executive notes that 83% of patients admitted through the emergency department with pneumonia had a blood culture test prior to the first dose of antibiotics. The most appropriate initial response is to:
   a. commend the staff for exceeding national averages.
   b. reprimand the staff for substandard care.
   c. institute staff training regarding appropriate pneumonia care.
   d. question the accuracy of the results.

- 61 -

55. Under the Joint Commission's National Patient Safety Goals, which of the following is generally acceptable as one of two required identifiers?
  a. Place of birth
  b. Date of birth
  c. Place of employment
  d. An armband taped to bedside stand

56. Which of the following is the most reliable indicator of increased employee engagement?
  a. Increased staff retention
  b. Increased job satisfaction (according to staff surveys)
  c. Decreased staff complaints
  d. Anecdotal reports of staff

57. When conducting SWOT analysis, which of the following is generally considered to be an external factor?
  a. Human resources
  b. Processes
  c. Physical resources
  d. Trends

58. Which of the following is an appropriate method for assessing the driving and restraining forces when doing strategic planning?
  a. Conducting a force field analysis.
  b. Establishing a task list.
  c. Conducting an events and causal factors analysis.
  d. Completing an affinity diagram.

59. A nurse executive whose responsibilities include acting as the company compliance officer finds what appears to be a long-standing pattern of fraudulent billing practices by the organization. Which of the following initial actions is most appropriate?
  a. Notify the appropriate regulatory agencies.
  b. Notify the board.
  c. Consult an attorney.
  d. Notify the police.

60. Which of the following is the best preparation for dealing with an internal disaster?
  a. Establishing a disaster management plan.
  b. Training staff in preventive measures.
  c. Advising staff to call 9-1-1 for crisis situations/disasters.
  d. Having regular fire drills.

61. When developing a nursing professional practice model, what would the nurse executive generally expect to find at the center of the model?
  a. Safety
  b. Care standards
  c. The patient and his/her family
  d. Professional values

62. Who or what is responsible for outlining a nurse's scope of practice?
    a. The American Nurses Association
    b. The American Nurses Credentialing Center (ANCC)
    c. Each state's Board of Nursing and Nurse Practice Act
    d. The American Academy of Nurse Practitioners

63. The primary benefit of instituting a yearlong <u>mentoring program</u> as part of new staff orientation is:
    a. increased staff retention.
    b. increased job satisfaction.
    c. decreased orientation costs.
    d. decreased need for supervision.

64. Which of the following types of research would require review by the Institutional Review Board?
    a. Research comparing the effectiveness of standard orientation program vs orientation plus mentoring
    b. Research involving the use of existing data without identifying subjects
    c. Research involving the evaluation of the effectiveness of different inservice delivery systems
    d. Research involving comparison of two different therapeutic approaches for the same disorder

65. When faced with the need to cut costly programs, which of the following is an example of <u>lateral thinking</u>?
    a. Reduce nursing and support staff and institute a hiring freeze.
    b. Reduce benefits for new hires and increase the use of part-time help.
    c. Develop a community-action plan to attract "sponsors" of various programs.
    d. Close satellite clinic sites and reduce onsite clinic hours.

66. When conducting literature research, which of the following has the most validity?
    a. An article in the *New York Times.*
    b. An article in *The Reader's Digest.*
    c. The transcript of a *60 Minutes (CBS)* television interview.
    d. An article in the *New England Journal of Medicine.*

67. When conducting internal research to determine if staff turnover is higher in the critical care unit than the general medicine unit, which of the following is the <u>dependent</u> variable?
    a. Turnover rate
    b. Staff assignments
    c. Staff gender
    d. Staff certification

      ↳ The research is trying to understand or explain

68. Which ethical system states that ethical decisions should be made to benefit the most people?
    a. Deontology
    b. Virtue
    c. Rights
    d. Act utilitarianism

69. Which aspect of outcomes evaluation refers to continuing treatment while still monitoring and evaluating?
    a. Improving
    b. Monitoring
    c. Sustaining
    d. Evaluating

70. When developing research questions, which of the follow is a complex hypothesis with multiple dependent variables?
    a. Senior nurses are less likely to support the expanding role of nurses than new graduates.
    b. Patients assigned a case manager have a more positive perception of nursing care than those without a case manager.
    c. Patients who are catheterized postoperatively develop more postoperative infections than those who are not catheterized.
    d. A structured plan for post-operative pain control is more effective than an unstructured plan in reducing patient complaints of pain and requests for pain medication.

71. For which of the following would qualitative research be more appropriate than quantitative research?
    a. Determining if an intervention decreases rehospitalization
    b. Evaluating patient response to two different medications
    c. Determining whether an electronic medication dispensing cart decreases medicine errors
    d. Assessing health beliefs of a particular culture

72. When conducting quantitative research with human subjects, at what point in the process must Institutional Review Board (IRB) approval be obtained?
    a. Immediately after identification of the problem
    b. Immediately after the collection of data
    c. Immediately before the collection of data
    d. Immediately before selection of the research design

73. What type of functioning is assessed by the CMS Minimum Data Set (MDS)?
    a. Nursing staff competency and accuracy
    b. Patient physical, psychological, and psychosocial functioning
    c. Administrative functioning, including Nurse Executive and Board of Directors
    d. Financial management, including budget and accounting practices

74. Which of the following is based on the strategic plan and provides performance measures in relation to the facility mission, vision statement, and goals/objectives?
    a. Pareto diagram
    b. Scattergram
    c. Dashboard
    d. Balanced scorecard

- 64 -

75. The hospital has collected and transmitted ORYX® data for 4 core measure sets. How many <u>non-core measures</u> are also required?

[handwritten: @ least 4 core measures OR a combo of fewer core measures + non-core measures.]

    a. 0
    b. 3
    c. 6
    d. 9

76. Considering the National Quality Forum's National Consensus <u>Standards for Nursing-Sensitive Care</u>, which of the following is classified as a <u>nursing-centered intervention</u> measure?

    a. Prevalence of pressure ulcers
    b. Falls resulting in injury
    c. Smoking cessation counseling for patients with heart failure
    d. Skill mix

77. If the nurse executive is collecting data for quality improvement by participating in the <u>voluntary consensus standards for nursing-sensitive performance</u>, how should data be collected and analyzed?

    a. By nurse
    b. By unit
    c. By department
    d. By institution

78. A unit supervisor states that she <u>enthusiastically</u> supports a new policy but does nothing to implement the needed changes and repeatedly makes excuses for delays. This communication style is:

    a. Assertive
    b. Passive
    c. Passive-aggressive
    d. Aggressive

79. According to Hackman's theory of group dynamics, which of the following is part of being "a real team?"

    a. Clear goal
    b. Shared task
    c. Open membership
    d. Moderate-sized group

80. The Board of Directors has proposed a change in benefits that will affect all full-time staff. What is the most appropriate method to communicate this change?

    a. Send emails
    b. Post notices
    c. Conduct staff meetings
    d. Meet one-on-one with affected staff

81. Which of the following is characteristic of successful coaching?

    a. Focusing on what the person is doing correctly
    b. Focusing on what the person is doing incorrectly
    c. Pointing out problem areas
    d. Providing a list of goals for the person

82. When an error or accident occurs in a just culture, who or what is usually initially considered at fault?
   a. The individual
   b. The system
   c. The administration
   d. The training

83. Which of the following is an example of horizontal violence?
   a. A senior nurse repeatedly interrupts a new graduate, stressing the new graduate's lack of experience.
   b. A staff member reports an act of negligence on the part of another staff member.
   c. A team leader tells the unit supervisor that she feels that one team member is in need of coaching.
   d. A staff member tells other staff that he believes a new policy is ineffective.

84. When considering space design, which of the following types of spaces is essential for family members and patients in a palliative care unit?
   a. Collector
   b. Mover
   c. Introspective
   d. Purpose

85. Which of the following is the best method of increasing staff participation in research?
   a. Providing a reward system
   b. Tying participation to pay scale
   c. Appealing to staff's professionalism
   d. Taking punitive action against those who don't participate

86. A staff member has proposed a new and promising procedure in the emergency department to decrease patient's length of stay. Which is probably the best initial way to proceed?
   a. Conduct a pilot study evaluating the change.
   b. Notify staff of the change in procedure.
   c. Ask for staff input into the change.
   d. Conduct small tests of the change.

87. Mandatory reporting of elder abuse is controlled by:
   a. state legislation.
   b. federal guidelines.
   c. certifying agencies.
   d. the institution.

88. According to the standard arbitration agreement of the American Arbitration Association, within what period of time, after written notification of a dispute, should the involved parties meet to try to reach an agreement?
   a. 10 days
   b. 30 days
   c. 60 days
   d. 90 days

- 66 -

89. Bundled payments provide revenue based on:
    a. fee for service.
    b. capitation.
    c. related diagnostic groups.
    d. expected costs of types of care.

90. The hospital has decided to outsource its electronic medical records (EMRs). The most common reason for outsourcing the EMR is:
    a. vendor expertise.
    b. cost savings.
    c. staff request.
    d. revenue increase.

91. Within the resource-based relative value scale (RBRVS) system, which of the following hospitals is most likely to receive the least payment for the same CPT codes from Medicare or HMOs?
    a. A large hospital in Manhattan, NY.
    b. A small hospital in Los Angeles, CA.
    c. A small hospital in Boston, MA.
    d. A large hospital in Bozeman, Montana.

92. During collective bargaining, union leaders stress the comparative-norm principle as part of salary negotiations. Based on this, the current salaries are probably:
    a. above the norm for similar institutions.
    b. approximately the same as similar institutions.
    c. No conclusion can be reached based on this information.
    d. below the norm for similar institutions.

93. When preparing for interest-based bargaining ("win-win") and contract negotiations, the nurse executive should expect to:
    a. share all bargaining information with union leaders.
    b. decide on a negotiation strategy.
    c. maintain an adversarial role.
    d. make major concessions.

94. The nurse executive makes decisions independently and strictly enforces rules of the organization. This type of organizational culture is best described as:
    a. bureaucratic.
    b. autocratic.
    c. consultative.
    d. *laissez-faire.*

95. While most unit supervisors have been supportive of changes that the nurse executive has instituted, one forceful unit supervisor has been a vocal opponent and has presented the nurse executive with a complaint signed by all members of the supervisor's staff. This is best described as an example of:
    a. coercion.
    b. brainwashing.
    c. insubordination.
    d. group think.

96. Which of the following is the most important element to include in a policy about whistle blowing?
    a. Processes that should be followed
    b. An outline of expected responses
    c. Protection from retaliatory action
    d. Timeframe

97. The time horizon for most operational budgets is:
    a. one month.
    b. three months.
    c. twelve months.
    d. five years.

98. When developing a budget, which of the following is an indirect cost?
    a. Wages
    b. Building depreciation
    c. Travel expenses
    d. Equipment costs

99. The organization purchased less expensive replacement equipment, but the equipment began to break down within a few months and had to be replaced again with a more expensive alternative. How would this additional cost be classified?
    a. Cost of quality
    b. Cost of poor quality
    c. Error-free cost
    d. Conformance costs

100. The revenue cycle for a patient begins with:
    a. services rendered.
    b. submission of claims.
    c. pre-registration/scheduling.
    d. registration.

101. When preparing to hire new personnel, the nurse executive prepares a job advertisement and application. Which of the following is an appropriate employment practice according to the US Equal Opportunity Commission?
    a. Advertisement states, "Ideal position for new graduates."
    b. Job application states," Do you have any disabilities?"
    c. Advertisement states, "Hispanic nurses needed to serve non-English speaking patients."
    d. Advertisement states. "Position requires fluency in both English and Spanish."

102. Which kind of analysis is used to compare costs of two different pancreatic cancer treatments that both result in average life extension of four months?
    a. Cost-benefit
    b. Cost-effectiveness
    c. Cost-utility
    d. Efficacy study

103. Which leadership concept is based on the idea that the leader should focus on staff strengths and not weaknesses or problems?
   a. Appreciative inquiry
   b. Servant leadership
   c. Situational leadership
   d. Pervasive leadership

104. If team members are primarily of medium maturity and are highly skilled but lack confidence in their abilities, the best leadership style according to the Hersey-Blanchard situational leadership model is:
   a. telling/ directing.
   b. selling/coaching.
   c. participating/supporting.
   d. delegating.

105. Activity based accounting enters:
   a. revenues when they are received and expenses when they are paid,
   b. revenues when they are earned and expenses when they are paid.
   c. revenues when they are projected and expenses when they are projected.
   d. revenues when they are earned and expenses as they are incurred.

106. The nurse executive believes that the hospital must invest in new software and technology as part of their strategic plan. The first step in this process is to:
   a. select an interdisciplinary team with knowledge about data needs and technology.
   b. identify system requirements for the organization.
   c. identify user needs.
   d. gain a commitment from the board for the financial outlay and the process of change.

107. The nurse executive wants to set up an organization-wide early warning system to screen patients for potential risks as a new risk management cost containment strategy. The system should identify:
   a. adverse patient occurrences and potentially compensable events.
   b. high risk patients and families.
   c. potentially high-risk procedures and compensable events.
   d. negligence and non-compliance with safe practices.

108. A rehabilitation hospital is considering utilizing telehealth for contract radiology diagnostic services. Which type of telehealth mode is most likely indicated?
   a. Real-time
   b. Store-and-forward
   c. Remote monitoring
   d. Hybrid of real-time and store-and-forward

109. The institution is planning to build a new ambulatory care center. Which layout is the most efficient in terms of time and effort for staff and patients?
    a. Single story building with the center and support services along a 400-foot corridor.
    b. Two story building 200 feet in length with the center on the first floor and support services on the second.
    c. Three story building 140 feet in length with the center on first and second floors and support services on the third.
    d. The center in one building and support services in another adjacent building.

110. The nurse executive is guiding efforts to develop competency validation for nursing skills. Which of the following is the best method to assess competency?
    a. True/False quiz
    b. Multiple choice quiz
    c. Laboratory demonstration
    d. Clinical observation/evaluation

111. With the accelerated rapid-change approach to quality improvement, the primary focus of teams should be on:
    a. generating and testing solutions.
    b. observing and reporting.
    c. analyzing and reporting.
    d. observing and evaluating.

112. The performance improvement model FOCUS (find, organize, clarify, uncover, start) is primarily used to:
    a. find solutions.
    b. analyze performance outcomes.
    c. identify problems.
    d. generate evidence.

113. When designing a performance improvement plan, the most important consideration is:
    a. its alignment with vision and mission statements and goals and objectives.
    b. the cost and resources needed for implementation.
    c. required performance measures.
    d. staff preference.

114. The nurse executive is monitoring performance improvement activities. Generally, how frequently should a written report of progress be issued?
    a. Daily
    b. Weekly
    c. Monthly
    d. Quarterly

115. The best strategy for writing a performance improvement plan is to:
    a. keep the plan brief and to the point, while stressing outcomes.
    b. outline the main points only.
    c. submit one section at a time for consideration.
    d. complete a comprehensive document explaining all details.

116. During negotiations, the nurse executive presents a plan. The union representatives agree to implement the plan although they prefer a different plan. This approach to negotiation is:
    a. Competition
    b. Accommodation
    c. Compromise
    d. Collaboration

117. A number of patient errors have occurred because of inadequate communication during hands-off procedures. Which of the following solutions is most likely to be effective?
    a. Provide an inservice about hands-off procedures.
    b. Increase disciplinary penalties for patient errors.
    c. Send emails to all appropriate staff.
    d. Implement use of the SBAR tool.

118. For facilities accredited by the Joint Commission, which of the following requires reporting as a sentinel event?
    a. An infant dies unexpectedly 12 hours after birth.
    b. A patient discharged from the psychiatric unit commits suicide 48 hours after discharge.
    c. A patient develops a hemolytic transfusion reaction because of blood group incompatibility.
    d. There is no requirement to report a sentinel event.

119. The nurse executive has received numerous complaints from community members about patient care policies and procedures. Which of the following is probably the best long-term solution?
    a. Respond to each complaint individually.
    b. Establish a patient/family advisory council.
    c. Refer the complaints to the staff.
    d. Conduct a community forum.

120. When delegating tasks to team members, the first step should be to:
    a. provide clear instructions.
    b. explain expected outcomes.
    c. assess team members' skills and availability.
    d. ask for volunteers.

121. Following a role-play exercise as part of disaster planning, which of the following is most important?
    a. Critical evaluation
    b. Brief time-out for all involved personnel
    c. Reassurance
    d. Debriefing period

- 71 -

122. The supervisor in the obstetrics department tells the nurse executive that the department nurses want to use standard care plans for outcomes identification. They feel that it would save time as patients have similar diagnoses and needs. Which response is most appropriate?

a. "That's a good plan."
b. "Let's institute that on a trial basis."
c. "That violates the ANA standards of practice."
d. "Absolutely not."

123. The state in which the nurse executive practices has passed a law requiring a licensed nurse-patient ratio of 1:5. The current ratio is 1:9 because nurse's aides assist the licensed nurses to provide care. What action is most likely necessary?

a. Recruit and hire new nurses.
b. Limit patient admissions.
c. Lay off nurse's aides, and recruit/hire new nurses.
d. Recruit and hire new nurses, taking money from the facility maintenance budget.

124. As the nurse executive and leader of a management team, which of the following can the nurse executive delegate?

a. Leadership
b. Discipline.
c. Planning and strategic goals.
d. Clinical observation.

125. Which of the following coding systems is used to define professionals licensed to provide services, and also to describe medical treatments and procedures?

a. Current Procedural Terminology (CPT)
b. International Classification of Disease (ICD)
c. Diagnostic-related group (DRG)
d. Universal billing (UB)

126. Global strategic planning usually establishes goals for up to:

a. one year.
b. 2 to 4 years.
c. 5 to 8 years.
d. 10 to 15 years.

127. One of the best ways for a nurse executive to advocate for others in the profession is to:

a. become active in state and national professional organizations.
b. exhibit competency.
c. blog.
d. publish articles in journals.

128. In a healthy work environment, "appropriate staffing" refers to:

a. the licensed nurse-patient ratio.
b. acuity staffing.
c. match of nurse competencies with needs of the patient.
d. specialized training for all staff.

129. The nurse executive exhibits altruistic behavior, listens effectively, and puts organization needs above personal. This is an example of:
    a. pervasive leadership.
    b. servant leadership.
    c. weak leadership.
    d. democratic leadership.

130. The best method for the nurse executive to build consensus and support for the strategic plan is to:
    a. update staff frequently.
    b. have a series of staff meetings explaining the strategic plan.
    c. include staff in planning.
    d. hire a consultant.

131. A nurse executive whose goal is to integrate cultural diversity and sensitivity into the workplace should ask staff members to focus on:
    a. intercultural exchange.
    b. self-awareness.
    c. experience.
    d. training.

132. Instead of meeting with unit supervisors and other staff in the administrative office or receiving written reports, the nurse executive has begun to meet with staff on the units, getting reports directly. This is a good example of:
    a. leadership visibility.
    b. servant leadership.
    c. pervasive leadership.
    d. a culture of transparency.

133. The organization has established both emergency and planned succession plans for the nurse executive position. Which of the following is most likely to be selected for emergency succession?
    a. An external consultant
    b. A retired nurse executive (5 years)
    c. A board member
    d. An internal candidate

134. In a crisis situation, the nurse executive remains calm, keeps her emotions under control and helps others to cope as well, sensing those who need extra support. The nurse executive is exhibiting:
    a. emotional intelligence.
    b. coaching.
    c. accessibility.
    d. visibility.

135. When planning to introduce a process improvement project with the goal of determining whether improved patient education results in fewer rehospitalizations, the initial step would be to:
    a. market the plan.
    b. outline educational content.
    c. obtain baseline data.
    d. establish specific goals.

136. What can the nurse executive do to create a common vision and facilitate change within the organization?
    a. Include all levels of staff across the organization in planning and implementation.
    b. Publicize the organization's mission and vision statements.
    c. Include nursing staff and physicians in planning and implementation.
    d. Ask for the staff's response to the organization's mission and vision statements.

137. Considering the dynamics of team building, what usually occurs during the initial interactions of a team?
    a. Members observe the leader to determine how control is exercised.
    b. Methods to achieve work are clarified.
    c. Members express willingness to support each other's goals.
    d. Members begin to define roles and develop relationships.

138. What is the primary purpose of drawing up a team contract?
    a. To ensure all members carry out expected duties.
    b. To provide a means of taking disciplinary action.
    c. To establish consensus about expectations of working within the group.
    d. To outline all of the duties the team is responsible for.

139. As part of a marketing plan, the nurse executive evaluates the costs of radio and television advertising. If a radio station charges $200 for a spot that reaches 200,000 people and a TV station charges $1000 for a spot that reaches 500,000 people, which is the least expensive per 1000 impressions (CPM)?
    a. Television ad
    b. Radio ad
    c. They are the same
    d. The data is inadequate to determine

140. Which trend is likely to most affect nursing practice in the next 10 years?
    a. Demographic changes
    b. Well-educated population
    c. Global economy
    d. Scientific advances

141. When applying for medical assistance through Medicaid, what period of retroactive coverage is allowed prior to the month the patient applies if the patient's condition would have warranted eligibility?
    a. No retroactive coverage is allowed
    b. One month
    c. Two months
    d. Three months

142. The nurse executive receives a call from another hospital verifying the work history of a nurse who had quit abruptly after drugs were found to be missing. She had informed the nurse executive that she was entering rehab for addiction. What should the nurse executive tell the person from the other hospital?

    a. That the nurse was suspected of being a drug user.
    b. That the nurse had been treated for addiction.
    c. That the nurse had worked at the hospital on the dates that the person indicated.
    d. That the other hospital should not hire the nurse.

143. The primary advantage of a computerized physician/provider order entry (CPOE) system is:

    a. faster initiation of treatment.
    b. decrease in medication errors.
    c. faster diagnosis of the patient.
    d. more efficient monitoring of patient's condition.

144. The 4 characteristics of Lean-Six Sigma are (1) long-term goals, (2) performance improvement, (3) utilization of improvement methodology, and (4):

    a. accountability.
    b. remediation.
    c. cost reduction.
    d. analysis.

145. When creating an organizational flow chart as a tool for quality improvement, a diamond-shape is used to indicate:

    a. input and output.
    b. a conditional decision.
    c. direction of flow.
    d. connectors with diverging paths.

146. Total Quality Management (TQM) focuses primarily on:

    a. cost-effectiveness.
    b. customer needs.
    c. organizational processes.
    d. organizational needs.

147. Events and causal factors analysis (E&CFA) is especially useful with:

    a. root-cause analysis.
    b. force field analysis.
    c. PDSA.
    d. CQI.

148. With process improvement projects, which of the following is a useful tool to manage schedules and estimate the time needed to complete tasks?

    a. Storyboard
    b. Pareto diagram
    c. Affinity diagram
    d. Gantt chart

149. The nurse executive uses medical jargon when talking to a group of patients, and they are confused about the content. Which element of communication is causing the confusion?
   a. Channeling
   b. Decoding
   c. Receiving
   d. Encoding

150. In the Health Communication Model (Northouse and Northouse), which element of communication refers to the setting and environmental conditions present during communication?
   a. Relationships
   b. Transactions
   c. Contexts
   d. Messages

Answers and Explanations

1. A: An Institutional Review Board must have a minimum of 5 members with at least one person a community member who is not affiliated with the organization and whose immediate family members are not affiliated with the organization. The other specific requirements are that one member be a "scientist" and one a "non-scientist." General requirements are that IRB members be knowledgeable and have the expertise required to make the necessary decisions. If human subjects include vulnerable populations (such as the elderly, children, or prisoners) then some members should be familiar with the issues these groups face.

2. D: The first step in strategic planning is to collect data and do an external analysis of customer needs in relation to regulations and demographics. The focus of strategic planning must be on development of services based on identified customer needs and then the marketing of those services. Other steps include:
   - Analyzing internal services and functions
   - Identifying and understanding key issues, including the strengths and weaknesses of the organization as well as potential opportunities and negative effects.
   - Developing a revised mission and vision statement that identifies core values.
   - Establishing specific goals and objectives.

3. A: The Joint Commission's Environment of Care requires management plans for six functional areas: safety, security, hazardous materials and waste, fire safety, medical equipment, and utilities. Management plans should include a risk assessment for each area, as well as plans for staff development to ensure compliance. Plans must also include emergency procedures and expected staff responses, detail programs for inspecting, testing, and maintaining the plans, and describe methods for collecting information and evaluating outcomes. Performance must be monitored and annual evaluations conducted.

4. B: Contemplation. The stages of change are:
   - **Precontemplation:** Informed about the consequences of problem behavior and has no intention of changing behavior in the next 6 months.
   - **Contemplation:** Is aware of costs and benefits of changing behavior and intends to change in the next 6 months but is procrastinating.
   - **Preparation:** Has a plan to initiate change in the near future (≤1 month) and is ready for an action plan.
   - **Action:** Modifies behavior. Change occurs only if behavior meets a set criterion (such as complete abstinence from drinking).
   - **Maintenance:** Works to maintain changes and gains confidence that he/she will not relapse.

5. D: This violates provision 1: The nurse treats all patients with respect and consideration, regardless of social circumstances or health condition. It is unethical to treat one group of patients differently than another simply because of their social circumstances (for example, being homeless or indigent). These patients should be evaluated and treated in accordance with the protocol established by the emergency department. This may vary from one

organization to another, but arbitrarily having their needs attended to after those of other patients is neither ethical nor medically justified.

6. B: Privileging follows the credentialing process and grants the individual authority to practice within the organization. Credentialing is the process by which a person's credentials to provide patient care are obtained, verified, and assessed in accordance with organizational bylaws. This process may vary from one organization to another. Members of a credentialing committee make decisions regarding credentialing and privileging, although some organizations use the Internet to verify credentials. Part of credentialing and privileging is determining what credentials are necessary for different positions, based on professional standards, licensure, regulatory guidelines, and accreditation guidelines.

7. C: Juran's 4 step quality improvement process involves the following four steps:
- **Defining** and organizing the project includes listing and prioritizing problems and identifying a team.
- **Diagnosing** includes analyzing problems and then formulating theories about their cause by root cause analysis. These theories are then tested.
- **Remediating** includes considering various alternative solutions and then designing and implementing specific solutions. This must be done while addressing institutional resistance to change. The processes should improve over time.
- **Holding** involves evaluating performance and monitoring the control system in order to maintain improvements.

8. B: Patients who are under 65 and newly disabled may apply for Medicare, with coverage beginning 24 months after the person begins getting SS or RRB disability benefits. The patient can, however, apply for Medicare part D between months 21 and 27 after receiving SS or RRB benefits. They should be advised to apply at month 21 to avoid delay in receiving Medicare D benefits. Patients who are already eligible because of disability and turn 65 can enroll for Medicare D during the period extending from the three months prior to turning 65 and the three months after.

9. A: Under the IRF PPS, patients are classified and placed into groups according to impairment categories. They are then grouped into case-mix groups (CMG) in which patients have similar motor functioning, age, and cognitive ability. These CMGs are further grouped into four tiers, depending on comorbidities. These groupings determine reimbursement. Adjustments may be made for short-term stays or transfers. Rates may be further adjusted according to geographic differences in wages and costs as well as numbers of low-income patients and presence of residency training programs.

10. D: Acuity-based staffing usually entails scoring the patients according to their needs for care. In some cases, computer programs are available to assist with this process. Those patients with the highest scores require the most nursing care, so staffing is adjusted to reflect these needs. With acuity-based staffing, the number of staff on a unit may fluctuate widely, depending on the type of patients. This type of staffing may require more flexibility than other models because more nurses may be assigned to serve as float nurses.

11. A: With Medicare, the benefit period, which began on admission to an inpatient facility, ends after the patient has been out of a medical facility for 60 days (including the day of discharge). Patients can have multiple benefit periods in one year but have to pay a hospital deductible for each benefit period. The first 60 days require no coinsurance but from days

62 to 90, the patient must pay a daily coinsurance charge. Hospitalization over 90 days requires use of lifetime reserve (for up to 60 days) or other form of payment.

12. C: **Indemnity insurance** pays in the form of predetermined payments for loss or damages rather than for healthcare service. **Liability insurance** pays damages for bodily injury or loss of property, such as from injury or damage resulting from unsafe conditions. **No-fault auto insurance** pays for injury/damages resulting from driving a car with coverage varying according to state regulations. **Accident and health insurance** pays for healthcare costs and may or may not, depending on the type of policy, include disability payments.

13. A: The purpose of stop-loss insurance, a form of reinsurance, is to protect an insurance company against excessive payments. Thus, the primary insurance may cover the first $150,000 of medical bills, and then the stop-loss insurance pays a percentage (usually around 80%) of the bills over that amount with the primary insurance paying the remainder (usually around 20%). Stop-loss is especially valuable for smaller, self-funded insurance plans.

14. B: **Bundling** occurs when an insurance plan negotiates a specific fee for a procedure, including all associated costs, and pays one bill. **Unbundling** occurs when a bundled agreement is dissolved, and the insurance plan pays separate bills (for the hospital, anesthesiologist, surgeon, etc.). **Fee-for-service** is the traditional billing method in which services are billed for separately. **Discounted fee-for-service** is similar to fee-for-service, except that reimbursements are discounted.

15. A: In a **market-driven approach** to healthcare, a market survey is conducted to determine current community needs. The survey should include the number and types of healthcare practitioners, the types of services offered, and the location so that the services offered are matched with the needs of the consumer. In a **provider-driven approach**, the providers make the major decisions about what services to provide and where. This depends on a variety of different considerations, including licensing laws and regulations regarding reimbursement.

16. D: In a targeted approach, the healthcare management focuses on the needs of a specific patient or a group of patients with similar problems. In this case, providing nutritional counseling directly to patients who are not adequately controlling their diabetes may improve outcomes by preventing complications and frequent hospitalizations, therefore reducing costs. These programs may set individual target goals as well, such as a specific weight loss or maintenance of a specific range of blood glucose levels.

17. C: The first step in developing a healthcare management program is to define the population needing to be served. This is usually derived from data regarding those with similar diagnoses, risks for complications, frequent need for clinical services, and/or high cost interventions. The program should then be developed with a specific goal, such as reducing costs or reducing complications, in mind. Barriers should be identified, as well as strategies to implement the plan and overcome those barriers. Finally, methods for measuring outcomes should be considered as well.

18. B: These criteria correspond to general subacute. Categories of subacute patients include:
- **Transitional subacute:** Estimated stay of 3 to 30 days and rehabilitation and/or nursing services 5 to 8 hours per day.
- **General subacute:** Estimated stay of 10 to 40 days and rehabilitation and/or nursing services 3 to 5 hours per day.
- **Chronic subacute:** Estimated stay of 60 to 90 days and rehabilitation and/or nursing services 3 to 5 hours per day.
- **Long-term transitional subacute:** Estimated stay of =/>25 days and rehabilitation and/or nursing services 6 to 9 hours per day. (Patients are often transferred to long-term care facilities.)

19. B: **Yes-no questions** are the easiest questions to quantify since this type of survey requires a choice between two categories, but they provide limited information. **Descriptive/information questions** often provide the most information, but results are difficult to quantify because each individual may answer questions differently. **Multiple-choice questions** must be designed carefully or clients may not find choices that reflect their opinions. These questions are also easy to quantify. **Rating scales** are used primarily to rate satisfaction or to indicate the level of agreement with a statement and—like multiple-choice questions—are easy to quantify.

20. A: There are 4 primary core criteria for credentialing and privileging:
- **Licensure:** This must be current through the appropriate state board, such as the state board of nursing.
- **Education:** This includes training and experience appropriate for the credentialing and may include technical training, professional education, residencies, internships, fellowships, doctoral and post-doctoral programs, and board and clinical certifications.
- **Competence:** Evaluations and recommendations by peers regarding clinical competence and judgment provide information about how the person applies knowledge.
- **Performance ability:** The person should have demonstrated ability to perform the duties to which the credentialing/privileging applies.

21. B: Denial or noncertification may result from extended hospitalization because PT or other services are not available on the weekend. Extended hospitalizations with cause, such as a myocardial infarction, are covered but may require concurrent authorization to notify the payor of changes in condition. A change in policy that takes place after services are rendered should not affect a case, as the effective policy is the one in place at the time of authorization. A client's death should result in termination of benefits rather than denial.

22. C: The Older Americans Act provides a wide range of home and community services for older adults, as well as respite services for family caregivers of older adults and children with special needs. OAA programs include support of senior centers, nutrition services, respite programs and long-term care planning. The OAA also supports health, prevention, and wellness programs for certain chronic conditions, which include Alzheimer's disease, diabetes and HIV/AIDS. They also promote self-management of chronic disease as well as the Healthy People 2020 initiative. The OAA is also involved with the protection of elder

rights by providing legal assistance, pension counseling and information services, and ombudsman programs.

23. D: An assisted living/custodial care facility is the appropriate placement for a client who has slight dementia but is otherwise medically stable and can ambulate and toilet independently. Unlicensed staff may assist patients in taking routine medications and can perform simple dry dressing changes. A home health nurse may be necessary if his needs become more complex. Clients may have home oxygen but should not require tracheal suctioning. Assisted living facilities are not usually appropriate for clients in need of rehabilitation or those who are more confused or disoriented because of safety concerns.

24. D: Unskilled care includes taking and reporting routine vital signs, assisting clients to take medications, assisting with personal care (bathing, applying lotions and creams, changing simple dressings), preparing meals, assisting with feeding, emptying drainage bags and measuring drainage, assisting with colostomy and ileostomy care, administering medical gases (after client has been stabilized), providing chest physiotherapy, assisting with stable tracheostomy care, and supervising exercises prescribed by a therapist. Performing simple range of motion (active and passive) exercises, and helping clients use assistive devices are also examples of unskilled care.

25. A: Once an action plan has been formulated, pilot testing should be conducted after determining the time frame, size of sample, and location(s). Then, the data from the pilot testing should be analyzed and the plan modified if necessary. With each modification, further pilot testing should be conducted until the action plan is ready for implementation. A timeline for implementation must be established with clear communication to all those involved and plans made for training and education.

26. C: When converting to an interoperable healthcare delivery system, the most important aspect to consider is the need for extensive training for all staff at all levels because the procedures that are currently paper-related must be modified and converted to a digital format. Standard terminology may need to be established or modified. Staff must be trained to input and retrieve information from the electronic system and safeguards must be established to prevent violations of confidentiality. Information retrievable over the Internet must be encrypted.

27. B: **Intermediate care** provides people with moderate assistance in activities of daily living and periodic nursing supervision for some activities, such as assistance with ambulation, grooming, and medications. Insurance companies usually do not pay for this level of care. **Custodial care/assisted living** provides people with assistance in performing basic ADLs, such as dressing and bathing. Insurance companies do not pay for this level. **Skilled nursing** provides maximal assistance with ADLs and also provide for daily supervision/care by a licensed professional. Insurance companies usually pay for this level of care. **Acute care** can include hospitals, rehabilitation services, inpatient rehabilitation centers, and transitional hospitals. Insurance companies should pay for this degree of care.

28. A: Steps to conflict resolution include:
First, allow both sides to present their side of the conflict without bias, maintaining a focus on opinions rather than individuals.
Encourage cooperation through negotiation and compromise.

Maintain the focus of the discussion, providing guidance to keep the negotiations on track and avoid arguments.

Evaluate the need for renegotiation, formal resolution process, or third party involvement. The best time for conflict resolution is when differences emerge but before open conflict and hardening of positions occur. The nurse must pay close attention to the people and problems involved, listen carefully, and reassure those involved that their points of view are understood.

29. C: The primary criterion for referral to a hospice program is the probability that death will occur within 6 months. Generally, hospice programs require a DNR order and a diagnosis of a life-threatening disease, but those alone are not sufficient, as those with longer life expectancies should be referred to palliative care programs instead. Severe intractable pain may be one problem hospice addresses, but pain can occur in patients who do not have a life-threatening disease.

30. C: Justice is the ethical principle that relates to the distribution of limited healthcare resources to members of society. These resources must be distributed fairly. This issue may arise if there is only one bed left and two patients in need of care. Justice comes into play when deciding which patient should stay and which should be transported to a different facility. The decision should be made according to what is best or most just for the patients and not colored by personal bias.

31. D: The **ADA** provides the disabled, including those with mental impairment, better access to the community and employment opportunities. Communities must provide transportation services for the disabled, including accommodation for wheelchairs. Public facilities (schools, museums, physician's offices, post offices, restaurants) must be accessible with ramps and elevators as needed. **EMTLA** prevents "dumping" of patients from emergency departments. **OAA** provides improved access to services for older adults and Native Americans, including community services (meals, transportation, home health care, adult day care, legal assistance, and home repair). **OBRA** provides guidelines for nursing facilities, such as long-term care facilities.

32. B: Presentation of only the 3 most cost-effective treatment options is a violation of the guidelines regarding informed consent, which include:
- Explanation of the diagnosis.
- Nature and reason for the treatment or procedure.
- Risks and benefits of the selected treatment.
- Alternative options (regardless of cost or insurance coverage).
- Risks and benefits of alternative options.
- Risks and benefits of not having a treatment or procedure.
- Providing informed consent is a requirement of all states.

While providing comparison information is not required, doing so does not violate informed consent protocols.

33. C: A **case mix group** (CMG) is a classification system based on the clinical characteristics of patients. **Resource utilization group** (RUG) is a classification system based on utilization of resources, with reimbursement tied to RUG level. The **Outcome and Assessment Information Set** (OASIS) is a data set used by home health agencies (HHA) to

measure outcomes and risk factors within a specified time frame. **Minimum data set** (MDS) contains elements to review for a comprehensive assessment of patient function. The MDS currently in use is MDS 3.0.

34. A: The primary purpose of sending an RFI to a variety of vendors is to help in the elimination and selection process. Topics for questions may include:
- History and financial status of company.
- Lists of current users of company's product.
- Information about system architecture.
- Hardware/software requirements.
- User support.
- Equipment support/maintenance.
- Ability of equipment to integrate with other systems.

Requests for information (RFI) are used early in system analysis to gather information from various vendors, often in conjunction with requests for proposal (RFP) and requests for quote (RFQ).

35. B: The first step to knowledge discovery in database (KDD) is data selection. Other steps include pre-processing (assembling target data set and cleaning data of noise), transforming data, data mining, and interpreting results. KDD is a method to identify patterns and relationships in large amounts of data, such as the identification of risk factors or effectiveness of interventions. KDD may utilize data perturbation, the hiding of confidential information while maintaining the basic information in the database, and data mining.

36. D: The American Recovery and Reinvestment Act (2009) (ARRA) included the Health Information Technology for Economic and Clinical Health Act (HITECH). Security provisions include:
- Individuals and HHS must be notified of a breach in security of personal health information.
- Business partners must meet security regulations or face penalties.
- The sale/marketing of personal health information is restricted.
- Individuals must have access to personal electronic health information.
- Individuals must be informed of disclosures of personal health information.

HITECH provides incentive payments to Medicare practitioners to adopt EHRs. Additionally, HITECH provides penalties in the form of reduced Medicare payments for those who do not adopt EHRs, unless otherwise exempted.

37. A: Switching to an acuity-based nursing care model to reduce overtime costs represents intelligent risk-taking because it stands a good chance of being successful, but failure is not likely to make things worse. Reducing nursing staff across the board in all departments is rarely a successful approach because the intensity of care needs often varies widely, increasing the risk of errors. Reducing support staff by 50% increases the burden on licensed staff and can result in costly problems. Hiring all part-time staff to avoid paying benefits often results in increased staff turnover and decreased engagement, both of which can be costly in the long-run.

38. D: **Social Exchange Theory** describes communication as an exchange system in which people attempt to negotiate a return on their "investment." **Social Penetration Theory** describes the manner in which people use communication to develop closeness to others, proceeding from superficial communication to more explicit self-disclosure. **Communication Accommodation Theory** explains why people alter their communication styles. Individuals may practice convergence or divergence. **Spiral of Science Theory** looks at the role that mass media has in influencing communication. It suggests that people fear isolation so they conform to public opinions as espoused by mass media and mute dissent.

39. B: Tracer methodology uses a selected patient's medical record as a guide to assess the continuum of care that a patient receives from admission to post-discharge. Tracer methodology uses the experience of this patient to evaluate the processes in place through documents and interviews. For example, if a patient received physical therapy, nursing and transport services, they would all be reviewed to determine how they received orders, carried out processes (including length of time and methods), and noted progress. Each step is traced and evaluated.

40. A: The primary purpose of knowledge management is to increase organizational effectiveness by ensuring that information reaches those who need it in an efficient and easily accessible manner. Knowledge includes that which is explicit and can be codified and transmitted through databases as well as tacit knowledge based on an individual's experience. An infrastructure must be in place to capture, create, and share content, including best practices, as well as expertise and experience (intellectual capital).

41. D: The Leapfrog Safe Practices Score assesses the progress a healthcare organization is making on 30 safety practices that Leapfrog has identified as reducing the risk of harm to patients. Leapfrog is a consortium of healthcare purchasers/employers and has developed a number of initiatives to improve safety. Leapfrog encourages voluntary public reporting and provides an annual Hospital and Quality Safety Survey to assess progress and release regional data. Leapfrog has instituted the Leapfrog Hospital Rewards Program (LHRP) as a pay-for-performance program to reward organizations for showing improvement in key measures.

42 A: Critical incident stress management (CISM) helps people cope with stressful events and in reducing the incidence of PTSD.
Defusing sessions: Very early, sometimes during or immediately after a stressful event to educate those actively involved about what to expect over the next few days and to provide guidance in handling feelings and stress.
Debriefing sessions: In 1-3 days after the incident and as needed for those directly and indirectly involved. People are encouraged to express their feelings and emotions. Six phases: introduction, fact sharing, discussing feelings, describing symptoms, teaching, and reentry.
Follow-up is done at the end of the process, usually after about a week.

43. C: Span of control is a business term that refers specifically to the number of subordinate staff a nurse executive (or any person) has and generally includes those subordinates the person personally supervises. Span of control is most important in a hierarchical organization where lines of authority are clearly delineated. The span of control may vary widely depending on the skills of the nurse and the skills of subordinates. Each subordinate, such as a unit supervisor, may also have a span of control.

44. B: National Quality Forum's safe practices include managing medications by implementing a computerized prescriber order entry (CPOE) system, using standardizing abbreviations, maintaining updated medication lists for patients, and including pharmacists in medication management to identify high alert drugs and dispense drugs in unit doses. Additional safe practices include considering patient's rights and responsibilities, managing information and care, preventing healthcare-associated infections, providing safe practices for surgery, and providing procedures and ongoing assessment to prevent site-specific or treatment-specific adverse events.

45. C: Discrete data, usually used to represent the count of something, are those that have a specific value and cannot be further quantified. Because the person creating the database and the person providing data are often different, eliciting the correct discrete data can pose problems, especially if the person providing data is not well versed in database design. One of the first steps to ensuring adequate data is to do a requirement analysis, which can involve eliciting information about data through case studies, interviews, focus groups, and observations.

46. A: Brainstorming is used to generate ideas about problems, processes, solutions, or other criteria in a short time frame. There are 5 primary steps:
Establish the purpose of and time frame for the brainstorming session.
Decide on a structured or unstructured approach.
Allow time for general discussion or individual thought.
List ideas according to the approach. Ideas may be written on a white board or flip chart or projected from a computer so that the group can look at the list.
Discuss items, clarify, and combine like items as the group agrees.

47. D: A **court order** authorizes disclosure of a patient's personal health information. In some cases, this court order may cover only restricted information rather than an entire health record. A **subpoena** is issued to advise a person that he or she must give testimony in court or in a deposition. A **subpoena *duces tecum*** is similar but requires that the person bring specific documents to court. A **warrant** authorizes an action, such as a search.

48. C: Workers' Compensation data are not available on a national basis. Criteria for data collection may vary from state to state along with state regulations, but even limited (statewide) data may provide an estimate of the frequency and severity of particular occupational injuries as well as their associated costs. The data may help guide the institution of work safety measures and development of safety training. Occupational illness data are less useful because injuries tend to be similar across industries while illnesses tend to show more variation.

49. D: When screening for medical cases for plaintiffs, the four necessary elements of negligence must be identified:
- **Duty of care:** The defendant had a duty to provide adequate care and/or protect the plaintiff's safety.
- **Breach of duty:** The defendant failed to carry out the duty to care, resulting in danger, injury, or harm to the plaintiff.
- **Damages:** The plaintiff experienced illness or injury as a result of the breach of duty.
- **Causation:** The plaintiff's illness or injury is directly caused by the defendant's negligent breach of duty.

50. B: Planning processes is an example of throughput. Components of Systems Theory include:Input:
Includes those things going into a system in terms of energy and materials, such as money, raw materials, effort, and time.
Throughput: Processes that transform the input, such as brainstorming, planning, meeting, and sharing resources and information.
Output: Resulting product, such as laws, rule, financial gain, materials, and programs.
Evaluation: Monitoring success or failure, such as through observation, surveys, and evaluations.
Feedback: Information derived from the product, such as accreditation reports.

51. A: Each case must be dealt with individually. If defined as a sentinel event, a root cause analysis that defines the problem through gathering evidence to identify what contributed to the problem must be performed. Once a root cause has been determined, an action plan that identifies all the different elements that contributed to the problem is recommended and instituted. The theory is that finding the root cause can eliminate the problem rather than just treating it. Thus, finding the source of an infection would be more important than just treating the infection.

52. C: The initial step in stakeholder analysis is to identify those stakeholders important to the organization by surveying key stakeholders and looking to see with whom they identify. Once a list is compiled, then surveys ask respondents to evaluate and rate the relative power of each of the stakeholders. Next, stakeholder mapping is usually done to show the relationships among the stakeholders. Stakeholders may be further classified as those who are primary (essential), secondary (non-essential), internal (within the organization), or external (outside the organization but interacting with it).

53. B: The Hospital Compare website allows people to compare up to 3 hospitals at a time. A search is conducted by zip code, city and state, or state alone. Results show distance from search parameter (such as distance from the zip code), availability of emergency services, and hospital type. Available information includes general information (address and types of services), patient survey results, timely and effective care in specified areas (heart attack, heart failure, pneumonia, surgical, ED, preventive care, and children's asthma), readmission complications and deaths, the use of medical imaging, Medicare payment, and number of Medicare patients.

54. C: The most appropriate initial response is to institute staff training regarding appropriate pneumonia care as the national average is 97%. While 83% represents less than optimal care, taking positive steps is more likely to bring about change than punitive steps. Data are provided at Hospital Compare as percentages, allowing comparison for up to 3 hospitals at a time. Data is shown for the selected hospitals as well as for state and national averages.

55. B: The Joint Commission requires two identifiers to ensure that the correct individual is receiving care and that the care is intended for that individual. Identifiers must be specific to the patient. The first identifier is usually the patient's name, often found on the wristband, and the second can be the birthdate, patient ID number, or telephone number. Birthplace is usually too non-specific as is place of employment. If an armband is used as an identifier, it

must be placed on the patient's body and cannot be simply placed at the bedside or taped to a bedside stand.

56. A: Increased staff retention is the most reliable indicator of increased employee engagement because it demonstrates a commitment to the organization, which is a critical element in engagement. Engaged employees are often more loyal and more productive. Employees can have high rates of job satisfaction without being engaged or actively trying to improve the organization, so surveys alone cannot measure engagement. Increased job satisfaction (with or without increased engagement) can lead to decreased complaints, but so can an intimidating environment in which employees are afraid to complain.

57. D: With SWOT analysis, strengths (S) and weaknesses (W) usually refer to internal factors, such as human resources, financial resources, physical resources, and processes. Opportunities (O) and threats (T) are more focused on external factors, which can include trends, sources of finances, rules and laws, the general economy, and national and international events. Because SWOT analysis evaluates the effect that internal and external factors have on work, it is sometimes referred to as an Internal/External Analysis. SWOT analysis is useful for both brainstorming and more in depth planning.

58. A: Force field analysis (Lewin) was designed to analyze both the driving forces (leaders, incentives, and competition) and the restraining forces (poor attitudes, hostility, inadequate equipment, and insufficient funds) for change. Steps include:
List the proposed change at the top and then create two subgroups (driving forces and restraining forces) below, separated by a horizontal line.
Brainstorm and list driving forces and opposed restraining forces. (When driving and restraining forces are in balance, this is usually a state of equilibrium or the *status quo*.)
Discuss the value of the proposed change.
Develop a plan to diminish or eliminate restraining forces.

59. C: Anyone in the position of potentially being a whistleblower needs to consult an attorney who specializes in whistle blowing before taking action. There are numerous federal and state laws and regulations about whistle blowing. Even more confusing is that they are often contradictory with different laws related to different professions and types of fraudulent actions. While whistleblowers are protected by many federal and state laws, the reality is that whistle blowing often results in loss of job, being ostracized or excluded, and/or civil action, so the person must fully understand the implications of their actions.

60. A: The best preparation for dealing with an internal or external disaster is to have a disaster management plan in place with all staff members thoroughly trained to understand their roles. The disaster plan should include procedures for fires, natural disasters (earthquakes, tornadoes, hurricanes, floods), chemical spills, communicable diseases, bomb threats, and utility failures. Emergency telephone numbers should be available and a telephone tree established. Plans for a command center should be outlined as well as lines of responsibility.

61. C: In most professional practice models, the patient/family is placed at the center of the model since the general goal of nursing is to provide excellent care for both the patient and his/her family. In some facilities, the practice model may focus on a slogan, such as "Patients first" or "Patient-centered care." Other aspects of the model are then developed to show how the caring environment is demonstrated. The professional practice model illustrates

Copyright © Mometrix Media. You have been licensed one copy of this document for personal use only. Any other reproduction or redistribution is strictly prohibited. All rights reserved.

the role and responsibilities of the nurse and usually includes emphasis on clinical quality care, professional development and professional values.

62. C: The state board of nursing and the Nurse Practice Act determines the nurse's scope of practice. Advance practice nurses, such as nurse practitioners or certified nurse specialists, are those who have completed additional education in an accredited nursing program (usually at a Master's level) and have received certification with a national certifying organization, like the American Nurse's Credentialing Center. The American Nurse's Association and the American Academy of Nurse Practitioners are professional organizations that may help to set standards but do not have legal authority to determine scope of practice.

63. A: A mentoring program is a critical element in improving staff retention. Some orientation programs are primarily classroom based with reviews of policies, procedures, and equipment. As a result, many nurses feel overwhelmed when orientation ends, especially new graduates who may lack the experience necessary to work autonomously. An ongoing mentoring program provides support for new nurses and the opportunity to benefit and learn from the experience of others. Formal mentoring programs usually establish one-on-one relationships rather than the more informal mentoring that occurs when one nurse assists another.

64. D: Research involving the comparison of two different therapeutic approaches for the same disorder would require review by the Institutional Review Board (IRB); an independent group that monitors research to ensure it is ethical. The Department of Health and Human Services, Title 45 Code of Federal Regulations, part 46 provides guidance for IRBs and outlines requirements for those involved in research. Institutions engaged in non-exempt research must submit an assurance of compliance document to the Office of Human Research Protection (OHRP), agreeing to comply with all requirements for research projects.

65. C: Vertical or rational thinking involves picking the "logical" solution to problems. In the case of the need to cut costs, this usually entails cutting back on staff or services. Lateral thinking looks at a problem from a different perspective and attempts to find a creative solution to a problem, considering all possible alternatives. When faced with the need to cut costs, the nurse executive utilizing lateral thinking might consider developing a community-action plan to attract "sponsors" of various programs. This is an innovative way to involve the community in cost-saving programs.

66. D: While all of these sources may, in fact, provide valid information, sources with the most authority are journals whose articles are peer-reviewed, such as the *New England Journal of Medicine*. Articles in the popular press undergo a much less rigorous review process. Besides considering the source, other important factors to consider when evaluating a source include the author's credentials, the strength of the thesis, how the article is organized, the evidence supporting or refuting the thesis, and the author's interpretation and analysis of the data.

67. A: The dependent variable is that which the researcher is trying to understand or explain, which in this case is the turnover rate. You can also think of the dependent variable as the presumed effect of something or some action. An independent variable is the presumed cause. In this type of research, besides looking at raw figures to determine the turnover rates in the two departments, the researcher would also attempt to identify other

independent variables (such as the assignments, staff gender, and staff certification) to determine if they could also affect the dependent variable or turnover rates.

68. D: The four major ethical decision making systems are as follows:

Act Utilitarianism	Ethical decisions are those that benefit the most people, regardless of personal feelings or laws. In Rule Utilitarianism, ethical decisions must take laws and fairness into consideration.
Deontology	When confronted with an ethical dilemma, people should adhere to obligations and duties.
Rights	Protects and supports the rights set up by society, such as those permitted by tradition or law. Individuals may also grant rights to others.
Virtue	When one's ethical decisions are questionable, then the person's morals and motivation (virtues) should be taken into account.

69. C: Outcomes evaluation includes the following:
- **Monitoring** occurs during the course of treatment and involves careful observation and record keeping that notes the patient's progress. Supporting laboratory and radiographic evidence is documented.
- **Evaluating** results includes reviewing records as well as current research to determine if the outcomes are within acceptable parameters.
- **Sustaining** involves continuing treatment, but also continuing to monitor and evaluate.
- **Improving** means to continue the treatment but with additions or modifications in order to improve outcomes.
- **Replacing** the treatment with a different treatment must be done if outcomes evaluation indicates that current treatment is ineffective.

70. D: A **complex hypothesis** predicts a relationship between an independent variable (a structured plan for post-operative pain control) and multiple dependent variables (perceptions of pain and requests for pain medication). Complex hypotheses are often more realistic than a **simple hypothesis,** which predicts the relationship between one independent variable and one dependent variable. A **directional hypothesis** predicts the direction of the relationship between the independent and dependent variable while a **non-directional hypothesis** predicts a relationship but not the direction.

71. D: While quantitative research is an objective empirical approach with clear steps, qualitative research is a much broader approach that allows researchers to generate theories and problems from subjective input, such as about health beliefs. Qualitative research can include field studies and historical research. Research is not data driven but instead depends on observation (as in field studies) and interviews. The researcher does not limit his analysis to relate to specific variables but attempts to find useful patterns in information.

72. C: IRB approval must be obtained immediately before beginning to collect any data. However, the research plan must be complete because this is what is reviewed by the IRB. They can approve, deny, or exempt the research proposal based on the content of the plan. Steps to the research process include:
- Identifying the problem and stating the purpose.

- Reviewing appropriate literature.
- Describing the theoretical framework.
- Defining relevant terms.
- Stating the hypothesis or hypotheses.
- Selecting the research design, including population and sample size.
- Obtaining IRB approval.
- Collecting data.
- Analyzing/Interpreting data.
- Publishing results/recommendations.

73. B: The CMS Minimum Data Set is a tool used to assess the physical, psychological, and psychosocial functioning of patients in long-term care facilities. The MDS applies to all long-term care facilities that are certified by CMS and must be used to assess all patients, even those not covered by Medicare or Medicaid. The tool helps to identify a patient's functional status and identify problems that must be addressed. Information is transmitted electronically to the state and then to the national CMS database.

74. D: The balanced scorecard (Kaplan and Norton) is based on the strategic plan and provides performance measures in relation to the mission and vision statement and goals and objectives. A balanced scorecard includes not only the traditional financial information but also data about customers, internal processes, and education. Each organization can select measures that help to determine if the organization is on track to meeting its goals. If the scorecard is adequately balanced, it will reflect both the needs and priorities of the organization itself and also those of the community and customers.

75. A: Hospitals must collect and transmit data for at least four core measure sets or a combination of fewer core measure sets and non-core measures. The only exception to this is free-standing children's hospitals, which must collect data on the core measure set, Children's Asthma care, and 9 non-core measures. This is because most core measure sets apply only to adults. Core measure sets include: Acute Myocardial Infarction, Heart Failure, Pneumonia, Perinatal Care, Hospital-Based Inpatient Psychiatric Services, Surgical Care Improvement Project, Hospital Outcome Measures, Venous Thromboembolism, Stroke, Emergency Department, Tobacco Treatment, Immunizations and Substance Abuse.

76. C: Nursing sensitive indicators are developed to determine the degree of influence that nursing provides, that is they establish correlation between nursing interventions and patient outcomes. The NQF's National Consensus Standards for Nursing-Sensitive Care has 3 framework categories with supporting measures:
- **Patient-centered** outcome measures: Falls, catheter-associated infections, ventilator-associated pneumonia, pressure sores, and surgical deaths.
- **Nursing-centered** intervention measures: Smoking cessation counseling for patients with acute MI, heart failure, and pneumonia.
- **System-centered** measures: Skill mix, nursing hours/patient, turnover, and practice environment scale.

77. B: If the nurse executive is collecting data for quality improvement by participating in the voluntary consensus standards for nursing-sensitive performance, data is usually collected and analyzed at the unit level unless the unit is so small that results point to an individual nurse. This is because it's important that the results be used to improve

processes rather than punish individuals. When reporting outcomes, the data should be reported at the institutional level.

78. C: The primary characteristic of a passive-aggressive communication style is a mismatch between what the person says and how the person acts. An assertive response would focus on reasons for agreement or disagreement and present them directly, while a passive response usually involves accepting direction with little response. This leaves decisions to others because of a lack of caring or a lack of confidence. An aggressive approach often includes criticism and even belittling of the other person's opinions in order to influence decisions.

79. B: Hackman's theory of group dynamics focuses on designing effective work groups and managing them appropriately. Effective work groups are productive with satisfied members who find meaning in the group participation. Hackman's conditions for effective group dynamics:
- Real team: Shared tasks and stable, understandable group membership.
- Direction: Clear directions and sequential goals.
- Structure: Varied tasks and moderate-sized group with members of appropriate skills and behavior.
- Support: Reward system in terms of information, equipment, recognition.
- Coaching: Availability of supportive expert coach when the need arises.

80. C: Because the change proposed by the Board of Directors affects many staff members, the nurse executive should conduct a staff meeting, which allows staff to express feelings about the proposed changes. Notices are one-sided communications because they don't provide for feedback and may be overlooked or cause resentment. Emails allow for exchange of idea, but responding to numerous emails with similar concerns can be time-consuming and impersonal. Meeting one-on-one with numerous staff is not an effective use of time.

81. A: Coaching can include training on specific skills, providing career information, and confronting issues of concern. While individual safety is the primary consideration, coaching should be done in a manner that increases learner confidence and ability to self-monitor rather than in a punitive or critical manner. Effective methods of coaching include:
Giving positive feedback, stressing what the student is doing right.
Using questioning to help the student recognize problem areas.
Providing demonstrations and opportunities for question and answer periods.
Providing regular progress reports so the student understands areas of concern.
Assisting the student to establish personal goals for improvement.
Providing resources to help the student master material.

82. B: It is common practice to blame the individual responsible for committing an error. However, in a just culture, the practice is to look at the bigger picture and to try to determine what characteristics of the system are at fault. For example, there may be inadequate staffing, excessive overtime, unclear orders, mislabeling, or other problems that played a role in the error being made. A just culture differentiates between human error, which results in consoling the person who committed the error; at-risk behavior, which results in coaching to prevent further error; and reckless behavior, which results in punitive action.

83. A: Horizontal violence is a form of bullying, most often directed at one or more individuals. When a senior nurse repeatedly interrupts a new graduate, pointing out his/her lack of experience, this is essentially belittling and intimidating behavior and may result in a lack of confidence on the new graduate's part. Horizontal violence can be physical (hitting, shoving), verbal (name calling, insulting, belittling, punishing), or non-verbal (rolling of eyes, inappropriate gestures).

84. C: **Introspective:** These areas are intended for peace and reflection although they may have high traffic. In some cases, this may be a chapel or a separate space where people can retreat into a quiet space. **Collector:** These are usually high traffic areas, such as waiting rooms, where the noise level may be quite loud. **Mover:** These are also high traffic and dynamic areas, such as hallways, where people move from one area to another. Noise levels are moderate. **Purpose:** These are areas with a specific purpose, such as treatment rooms, so the traffic flow is usually moderate, and noise level can vary.

85. A: The best way to increase staff participation in research is to provide a reward system of some type, such as recognition, credit for continuing education, increased pay, and/or increased responsibility. Tying participation to pay scale and taking punitive action against those who don't participate are both non-productive options because people may feel forced to participate and/or become resentful and passive aggressive. While appealing to professionalism is a good strategy for a few people, it is unlikely to be successful without some form of a reward system.

86. D: Conducting small tests of change, such as using the new procedure for one shift and then seeking feedback before conducting further small tests of change, is probably the best way to proceed because it is non-threatening to those who are resistant to change and can provide valuable feedback. If the initial test is successful, then the next test may be conducted for one or two days. In some cases, asking for volunteers to participate in the new procedure may be helpful. A number of small tests for change may be linked with increasing participation until enough information is gained for a full pilot study or for implementation.

87. A: Each state has established its own rules for mandatory reporting, including who must report and under which circumstances. While there are similarities, there are also crucial differences, so the nurse executive should be aware of the appropriate state regulations. In all states, healthcare providers and teachers, as well as some allied health professionals (such as social workers), are considered mandatory reporters of child abuse, elder abuse, and domestic violence. Reports may need to be made to different state agencies. In addition, abuse may be defined differently depending on the state.

88. B: While arbitration agreements can be customized for any organization, the standard arbitration agreement of the American Arbitration Association states that the parties involved in a dispute should meet to try to resolve the issue within 30 days after written notice of the dispute is received. If the parties cannot reach an agreement within 30 days, then the dispute must be resolved through arbitration. The request for arbitration must be made within 2 years from the time the party with the complaint was aware of the problem/dispute.

89. D: Bundled payments are based on expected costs associated with episodes of care; so, for example, one payment is made to cover hospitalization, physician care, and other required services and then the money is dispersed to each care provider. Defining an episode of care can be quite complex because all of the associated costs, services and providers must be identified beforehand and then it is necessary to determine how much reimbursement each party will receive.

90. A: The most common reason for outsourcing is vendor expertise although cost savings is also often a significant benefit. Studies show that patient care services are more often outsourced than IT services. In most cases of outsourcing, a contractual agreement outlines each party's responsibilities although some joint venture agreements occur. In most cases it is the vendor, rather than the institution, that assumes both the risks and rewards associated with providing the service. Services commonly outsourced include dialysis, anesthesia, laboratory and diagnostic testing, hospitalist services, and emergency department management.

91. D: The large hospital in Montana is most likely to receive the lowest payment from Medicare and HMOs because payment is based on physician work (52%), expense of practice (44%), and malpractice costs (4%). A relative value is assigned based on geographic location. Because overhead costs and costs for services tend to be higher in large cities such as New York, Los Angeles, and Boston, payment for the same CPT codes may be higher there than in more rural areas, like the hospital in rural Montana.

92. D: The comparative-norm principle states that workers in the same industry/organization or with the same bargaining relationship should have similar salaries, often referred to as the industry standard. Because the union leaders are stressing this principle, it means that the current salaries are probably below the norm for similar institutions. In situations where salaries are higher than the industry standard, it is more likely that the administration may refer to the comparative-norm principle in arguing against salary increases.

93. A: Interest-based bargaining ("win-win") is based on sharing of all bargaining information in order to reach a consensus and find solutions. IBB stresses the issues at hand and looks for solutions to current and future problems rather than focusing on past experiences. In IBB, both sides recognize that they share some of the same interests even though their approaches may be different. They each recognize that both parties may need to make some concessions so that each side can get a part of what they want.

94. B: In an autocratic culture, the nurse executive makes decisions independently and strictly enforces rules. Staff members often feel left out of process and may not be supportive. This type of leadership is most effective in crisis situations where fast decisions are necessary, but this leader may have difficulty gaining the commitment of her staff, who may feel marginalized. Additionally, because the leader does not want input from others, creative or new solutions to problems may be overlooked. The autocratic leader may be viewed as bossy and dictatorial, which can be undermining to staff morale.

95. D: This is an example of **group think,** which occurs when members of a group defer to one idea and support it collectively without giving consideration to its merits. This often occurs when a forceful leader takes a position and convinces others to support the position. **Coercion** involves forcing others to do something against their will, usually with threats.

Brainwashing is an extreme form of mind control in which the person is no longer able to make rational independent decisions. **Insubordination** involves disobedience and/or misconduct of some type in refusing to respect authority.

96. C: The most important element to include in a policy regarding whistle blowing is the protection of the reporting staff member from retaliatory action as many people are fearful that they will lose their job or be otherwise punished. A whistleblower policy should clearly outline the process for reporting concerns and should ensure that action will be taken to investigate the concern within a specified timeframe.

97. C: The time horizon is the actual time covered by the budget cycle. While this can be set for any timeframe, most operational budgets have a time horizon of 12 months. The operational budget is used for daily operations and includes direct and indirect expenses, such as salaries, education, insurance, maintenance, depreciation, debts, and profit. The budget has 3 elements: statistics, expenses (including losses), and revenue. A budget is balanced when expenses are covered by revenue.

98. B: Indirect costs are the overhead costs associated with facilities and administration, like building depreciation, because they are not specifically identified with a particular service or department. Direct costs are easily tied to a specific function, department or service and include salaries and wages, benefits, supply and equipment costs, travel expenses, consultant fees, contract costs, and costs of patient care. Both indirect and direct costs must be calculated and/or estimated as accurately as possible during budget planning.

99. B: The cost of poor quality (COPQ) is a cost that would not occur if there were no quality issues. COPQ is one factor in cost of quality (COQ), which includes costs associated with identifying and correcting errors, making errors, and identifying defects or failures in processes or planning. COPQ may be direct, such as the costs associated with purchasing new equipment, or indirect, such as the costs in terms of lost efficiency and time. Indirect costs are more difficult to quantify but may be substantial.

100. C: The revenue cycle for a patient begins when the patient is pre-registered or scheduled for care and ends when all revenues have been received, leaving a zero balance. Managing the revenue cycle efficiently is critical to maintaining a balanced budget. On pre-registration, all of the patient's demographic and insurance information, such as policy, benefits, and the necessary authorizations for care, must be obtained. After services are rendered, claims must be submitted promptly with the correct coding so that payment is not delayed. Patients must be billed for non-covered services, and all services should be reviewed and deemed appropriate by utilization review.

101. D: "Position requires fluency in both English and Spanish" focuses on the skills needed but does not limit applicants to one group, such as "Hispanic nurses." Employers are specifically prohibited from asking people if they have a disability although they can ask if they require accommodations. Advertising a job for "new graduates" may give the appearance of age discrimination since new graduates are usually under age 40. Employers cannot discriminate on the basis of age (≥40), disabilities, gender, race, religion, pregnancy, or genetic information.

102. B: A cost-effective analysis measures the effectiveness of an intervention rather than only the monetary savings. For example, about 2 million nosocomial infections result in

- 94 -

90,000 deaths and an estimated $6.7 billion in additional health care costs each year. From that perspective, decreasing infections should reduce costs, but there are also intangible savings (like prevention of human suffering) and it can be difficult to place a monetary value on those. If each infection adds about 12 days to a patient's stay in the hospital, then if five fewer patients suffered from a reduction in infection would be calculated:
5 x 12 = 60 fewer patient infection days.

103. A: Appreciative inquiry is a leadership concept that focuses on a person's strengths rather than weaknesses. It proposes that all questions suggest a bias because people tend to look in the direction of the question. For example, if someone asks "What is the problem?" then people will automatically assume a problem exists rather than looking more broadly and openly. The underlying philosophy is that belief influences action, inquiry results in change, words carry impact beyond simply meaning, actions are guided by future projections, and change needs positive efforts.

104. C: According to the Hersey-Blanchard situational leadership model, if team members are primarily of medium maturity and are highly skilled but lack confidence (M3), the best leadership style is participating/supporting (S3). Situational leadership proposes that the type of leadership needs to meet the needs of the team members or group. So those with low levels of maturity (M1) need telling/directing leadership (S1). Those with medium levels of maturity but limited skills (M2) need selling/coaching (S2), and those with high levels of maturity (M3) need delegating leadership (S4)

105. D: Activity-based costing (ABC) system is an accounting system focused on the costs of resources necessary for a process or service. Traditional accounting (a cash basis system) enters revenues when they are received and expenses when they are paid, so that revenues and expenses are not necessarily related. ABC is an accrual system, and does the accounting differently. Revenues are entered when they are earned and expenses as they are incurred so that revenues and expenses are more closely tied. The basic formula for ABC is to divide the total output into total cost to arrive at a unit cost.

106. D: The first step in investing in new hardware and software is to gain a commitment from the board for the financial outlay and the process of change it will entail. Evaluating hardware and software is a time-intensive process, so beginning as speculation is not productive. Once a commitment is made, then an interdisciplinary team should be formed, system requirements and user needs identified, the current system assessed, and vendors evaluated. The next step will be to evaluate and compare different software programs and hardware. The last steps are to negotiate a contract and implement the new system.

107. A: For risk management purposes, an organization-wide early warning system should be in place to screen patients for potential risks and to identify the following:
Adverse patient occurrences (APOs): Those unexpected events that result in a negative impact on the patient's health or welfare.
Potentially compensable events (PCEs): APOs that may result in legal claims against the organization because of the negative impact on the patient's health or welfare.
If the organization has set up a method to quickly identify and manage problems, the risks may be minimized.

108. B: Telehealth is increasingly used for radiology diagnostic services because the radiologist can easily read the films remotely on a computer and transmit the report back to

the facility. There are several different telehealth modes that can be utilized: **Store-and-forward** occurs when files are transmitted and stored until the report is sent. This is the most commonly used model for this type of service. Turn-around time varies but is usually within 48 hours, depending on the contractual agreement. **Real-time telehealth** involves video-conferencing and live consultations between staff and patients. **Remote monitoring** is used to monitor cardiac status, nocturnal dialysis, and other health conditions.

109. B: Generally speaking, having all the services in one area is most efficient, so maintaining both the center and support services in one building and on one floor is ideal, if possible. However, once people have to walk more than about 250 to 300 feet, it becomes more efficient to take an elevator to a second floor (in terms of time and energy spent walking from one area to another). In this case, the best option is likely the two-story building that is 200 feet in length.

110. D: While true/false and multiple choice quizzes may be helpful in assessing knowledge, especially after nurses have taken classes, knowledge and nursing skills are not always the same. Laboratory demonstrations are helpful as part of learning activities, but the anxiety level of participants may be different because there is no real danger of doing harm. The best method to assess competency is to observe the nurse in actual clinical situations and use an evaluation form/checklist during observations to ensure that competency standards are met.

111. A: The accelerated rapid-cycle change approach is a response to rapid changes in healthcare delivery and radical reengineering. There are 4 areas of concern:
Models for rapid-cycle change: The goal is doubling or tripling the rate of quality improvement by modifying and accelerating traditional methods. Teams focus on generating and testing solutions rather than analysis.
Pre-work: Assigned personnel prepare problem statements, graphic demonstrations of data, flowcharts, and literature review. Team members are identified.
Team creation: Rapid action teams (known as RATs) are created to facilitate rapid change.
Team meetings and work flow: Meetings/work done over 6 weeks.

112. C: Find, organize, clarify, uncover, start (FOCUS) is a performance improvement model that, by itself, is an incomplete process and is primarily used as a means to identify a problem rather than a means to find the solution. FOCUS is usually combined with PDSA (FOCUS-PDSA), so it becomes a 9-step process, but beginning with FOCUS helps to narrow the focus, resulting in better outcomes. Steps:
Find: Identify what's working and what isn't.
Organize: Identify those people who understand the problem and can act.
Clarify: Brainstorm solutions.
Uncover: Analyze reason for problem.
Start: Determine where to begin the change process.

113. A: Designing a performance improvement plan includes strategic planning for organization-wide participation and collaborative activities, which may be department/discipline specific or interdisciplinary. The plan must be consistent with vision and mission statements and goals and objectives. All performance activities must be referenced to the specific strategic goals or objectives that are part of the mission and vision statements. If there is a disparity, the vision and mission statements may need to be adjusted or the focus of the improvement activities changed.

114. C: Process improvement activities should be reported on regularly, usually monthly, both in written form and in presentations at team and management meetings. Daily or weekly written reports may not show a lot of change because of the short timeframe and because analyzing data may be time-consuming. Monthly reports at a meeting of directors/managers can then be disseminated through staff, team, and department meetings. A calendar should be generated based on a proposed timeline with regular meetings times established.

115. D: The written plan may vary depending upon its purpose. It may be brief if it is intended primarily as a teaching tool to guide staff, but if it is used as a tool for implementation, it should be a comprehensive written document that outlines in detail all of the different aspects of the performance improvement plan. A detailed plan must include a statement of commitment, a clear outline of authority and responsibility, an explanation of the infrastructure and outline of the flow of information. The goals and objective of the plan should clearly relate to strategic goals and objectives.

116. B: **Accommodation:** One party concedes even though the losing side may gain little or nothing, so this approach is most useful when there is a clear benefit to one choice. **Competition:** One party wins and the other loses, such as when parties are unwilling to compromise. To prevail, one party must remain firm, but this can result in conflict. **Compromise:** Both parties make concessions to reach consensus, but this can result in decisions that suit no one, so compromise is not ideal. **Collaboration:** Both parties receive what they want, often through creative solutions, but collaboration may be ineffective with highly competitive parties.

117. D: The SBAR tool is a systematic method of communication that is especially useful during hands-off procedures because it helps the nurse to organize information and present it clearly. Hands-off procedures should be documented and adequate time allowed for communication, including questions from the receiving party. SBAR:
(S) Situation: Overview of current situation and important issues.
(B) Background: Important history and issues leading to current situation.
(A) Assessment: Summary of important facts and condition.
(R) Recommendation: Actions needed.

118. D: The Joint Commission does not require reporting of sentinel events but encourages healthcare organizations to voluntarily report these events. The Joint Commission publishes a list of reviewable sentinel events, such as anything resulting in an unexpected death or severe physical or psychological injury, but each organization can, in addition, establish its own list of sentinel events. Reporting sentinel events contributes to TJC database, allows the organization to consult with TJC staff, and demonstrates openness.

119. B: The best long-term solution would be to establish a patient/family advisory council so that community members can have some input into policies and gain a better understanding of the organization and hospital staff can become more aware of community concerns. In a large institution, there may be a general patient/family advisory council that discusses the institution as a whole in addition to patient/family advisory councils for specific units or departments, such as pediatric oncology.

120. C: The first step in delegating tasks to team members is to assess the skills and available time of the team members, determining if a task is suitable for an individual. Then, the task should be assigned with clear instructions that include explanation of objectives and expectations, including a timeline. Progress should be monitored but not micromanaged to ensure that tasks are completed properly. Because the leader is ultimately responsible for the delegated work, mentoring, monitoring, and providing feedback and intervention as necessary during this process is a necessary component of leadership.

121. D: The point of a role-play exercise is for people to learn and to recognize areas of strength and weakness. An essential element of role play is the debriefing period that follows the conclusion of the exercise. All participants should be encouraged to express their feelings and opinions about the exercises. The discussion and questions that arise can be helpful in improving performance. Those conducting the exercise can note the positive and negative observations they made without singling out individuals.

122. C: Outcomes assessment as part of the care plan must be individualized, so using standard care plans is precluded even though they may be referred to as a guide. Nurses should never assume that all patients are exactly the same in terms of care needs or expected outcomes, and care plans should be updated regularly, reflecting any changes in patient condition. The ANA's Standards of Practice for All Registered Nurses, Standard 3, states that the nurse develops an individualized plan for expected outcomes.

123. C: The reality is that in states in which the legislature has established mandatory licensed nurse-patient ratios, allied help, such as nurse aids are typically laid off as new nurses are hired because of budget constraints, but this often leaves licensed nurses burdened with needing to provide basic care, such as bathing and changing linen, while also managing care that require professional expertise. Some states have taken a different approach, such as requiring staffing plans. New Jersey requires hospitals to post their nurse-patient ratios publically.

124. D: Clinical observations can be a delegated task, but the other tasks should be the responsibility of the leader. While delegation of tasks in central to working in teams, determining non-delegated tasks is also necessary. Not every task can be delegated because those issues related to strategic planning and management must be retained by the leader. Non-delegated tasks include leadership, the monitoring process, discipline, strategic goals and planning, communication and availability for consultation, and direction of the final outcomes assessment.

125. A: Coding systems include:
- **Current procedural terminology (CPT):** Developed by the American Medical society and used to define those licensed to provide services and to describe medical treatments and procedures.
- **International Classification of Disease (ICD):** Developed by the WHO and used to code for diagnosis.
- **Diagnostic-related group (DRG):** Used to classify a disorder according to diagnosis and treatment.
- **Universal billing (UB):** Used to describe hospital services, including demographic information, diagnostic and treatment codes, and charges for services.

126. D: Global strategic planning requires that an organization look at needs of the organization, community, and customers and establish goals for not only the near future (2-4 years) but into the extended future (10-15 years). Strategic planning must be based on assessments, both internal and external, to determine the present courses of action, needed changes, priorities, and methodologies to effect change. The focus of strategic planning must be on development of services based on identified customer needs and then the marketing of those services.

127. A: While all nurse executives should exhibit competency, and blogging and publishing are worthwhile, the best way to advocate for others in the profession is to become active in state and national professional organizations. These organizations influence legislation that affects the profession and often sets standards of practice. The nurse executive can participate by giving conference presentations and serving on committees or assuming a leadership role. An organization of special interest is the American Organization of Nurse Executives, which is a subsidiary of the American Hospital Association.

128. C: In a healthy work environment, there should be a match between the nurse competencies and the needs of the patient so that the patient is able to receive optimal care and the nurse feels confident in his/her abilities to provide that care. Other aspects of a healthy environment are skilled communication, true collaboration, effective decision-making, meaningful recognition, and authentic leadership. All staff should work collaboratively to make changes that result in a healthy work environment.

129. B: A nurse executive who exhibits altruistic behavior, listens effectively and puts organization needs above personal is exhibiting servant leadership, a concept developed by R.K. Greenleaf in 1970. The servant leader focuses on serving the organization and others and is able to influence and guide other through persuasion and reason rather than coercion and recognizes the contributions of all staff members. The servant leader especially has empathy toward others and has personal self-awareness, recognizing personal strengths and weaknesses.

130. C: The best method for the nurse executive to build consensus and support for the strategic plan is to include staff in the planning phases because this approach is almost always better than trying to convince people after the fact, regardless of the merits of the plan. Once the strategic plan is finalized then the staff should be updated frequently and staff meetings held to explain and discuss the strategic plan and changes that will be needed to implement the plan.

131. B: A nurse executive striving to integrate cultural diversity and sensitivity into the workplace should ask staff members to begin with self-awareness by assessing their own cultural perspectives and potential biases. It is incumbent on staff to ensure that all patients/families receive equal quality care but with delivery of care tailored to meet the individual needs of the patients. This begins with asking staff to assess their own attitudes and open discussion about differences to help people to gain self-awareness and determine if their ideas are stereotypical and/or based on lack of knowledge.

132. A: Meeting on the units with staff supervisors and getting reports directly is a good example of leadership visibility because, by taking the time to go to the units, the nurse executive is being seen by other staff members, and this gives the appearance that the leader is involved and taking an active interest in the work of others in the organization.

Efforts to increase visibility also provide the opportunity for the nurse executive to make more direct observations and to interact more with staff.

133. D: An internal candidate is usually selected for emergency succession because of the need to immediately step into the position and to be familiar with the organizational structure and current demands of the position. The chosen candidate usually fulfills the position on a temporary basis until planned succession can occur. Plans for succession should always be in place so that transitions are not disruptive to the organization. Planned succession may focus on both internal and external candidates, depending on the needs of the organization.

134. A: The nurse executive is exhibiting emotional intelligence by processing emotional matters while controlling personal emotions and helping others to control theirs. The model (Salovey and Mayer) includes:
Ability to perceive emotions: To look at a person's facial expression and to understand and perceive that person's emotions.
Ability to use emotions: To use emotions and changing moods to improve problem solving and thinking processes.
Ability to understand emotions: To comprehend and be sensitive to the subtleties of emotion.
Ability to manage emotions: To control emotions of the self and others.

135. C: This process improvement plan should result in quantifiable results, so the first step is to obtain baseline data so that variances can be traced as new data are collected. Baseline data is usually obtained for a prescribed period of time—generally one month—with the basis for alerts predetermined so that once data triggers a variance alert, then statistical analysis must be completed to determine the relevancy of the variance, the probability of it having occurred by chance, in order to determine if the variance has statistical significance.

136. A: Creating a common vision and facilitating change require considerably more than publicizing or asking for comments on mission and vision statements because if staff don't share the vision, then making changes will be very difficult. The best method to create a common vision is to include all levels of staff across the organization, nursing and non-nursing, in planning and implementation. The nurse executive can build consensus through discussions, inservice, and team meetings to bring about a convergence of diverse viewpoints. Creativity should be encouraged and a vision statement should support that common vision that is accessible to all staff.

137. D: During **initial team interactions**, members begin to define roles and develop relationships. Other dynamics then become evident:
Power issues: Members form alliances and observe the leader to determine who controls and how control is exercised.
Organizing: Methods are clarified, and team members begin to work together toward a common goal.
Team identification: Interactions often become less formal and members are more willing to help and support each other to achieve goals.
Excellence: This develops through a combination of good leadership, committed team members, clear goals, high standards, external recognition, spirit of collaboration, and a shared commitment to the process.

138. C: The primary purpose of a team contract is to establish consensus about expectations of working with the group. Contracts include:

Roles: Delineate specific responsibilities of each team member.

Discussion: Outline manner in which discussion is to be held (agenda driven, Robert's rules, open discussion).

Time: State amount of time members must commit to team activities and meetings.

Conduct: Clarify acceptable behavior parameters for individuals and the group.

Conflict resolution: Agree upon triggers and methods for conflict resolution.

Reports: Clarify types of reports, timeline, and responsibility for preparing the reports.

Consequences: Identify consequences for Failure to follow the contract.

139. B: The CPM for the radio ad is $1.00 per 1000 impressions and the CPM for TV ad is $2.00 per 1000 impressions, so the radio add is the least expensive with the TV add costing twice as much to reach the same number of people. CPM, cost per *mille* (thousand), is a standard method of calculating advertising rates. At $200 for 200,000 impressions: 200/200 = $1.00 to reach 10000. At $1000 to reach 500,000: 1000/500 = $2.00 to reach 1000.

140. A: While all of these trends will impact nursing, the most immediate impact is likely to result from demographic changes, including the "graying" of the population with a fifth of the population over age 65 by 2020. The emphasis on preventive medicine and care of chronic disease will increase to meet changing needs. Additionally, the population is becoming more ethnically diverse, and t his is reflected in nursing school enrollments. Nursing students are also becoming older as people enter nursing as a second career, often while juggling family responsibilities.

141. D: Patients applying for medical assistance through Medicaid can receive 3 months of retroactive coverage if the patient's condition would have warranted eligibility. Medicaid is a combined federal and state welfare program authorized by Title XIX of the Social Security Act to assist people with low income with payment for medical care. This program provides assistance for all ages, including children. Older adults receiving SSI are eligible as are others who meet state eligibility requirements. The Medicaid programs are administered by the individual states, which establish eligibility and reimbursement guidelines, so benefits vary considerably from one state to another.

142. C: This is a legal and ethical dilemma because the nurse executive may suspect that the nurse took drugs from the hospital, but the nurse quit and was not fired, there was no proof the nurse had taken the drugs, and the nurse has a right to privacy regarding treatment for addiction. From a legal standpoint, the nurse executive should only verify the person's employment but refrain from giving a positive or negative recommendation and should not share unproven suspicions.

143. B: Computerized physician/provider order entry (CPOE) are clinical software applications that automate medication/treatment ordering, requiring that orders be typed in a standard format to avoid mistakes in ordering or interpreting orders. CPOE is promoted by Leapfrog as a means to reduce medication errors. About 50% of medication errors occur during ordering, so reducing this number can have a large impact on patient safety. . Most CPOE systems also contain a clinical decision support system (CDDS) so the system can provide immediate alerts related to patient allergies, drug interactions, duplicate orders, or incorrect dosing at the time of data entry.

144. C: Lean-Six Sigma is a method that aims to reduce error and waste within an organization through continuous learning and rapid change, so one of the primary characteristics is cost reduction through quality increase, supported by statistical evaluation of the costs of inefficiency. Goals and strategies to reach the goals should be in place for periods of 1 to 3 years. The underlying belief system should be focused on performance improvement at all levels in the organization, and methods for process improvement, such as PDSA, should be utilized.

145. B: A flow chart is a tool of quality improvement and is used to provide a pictorial/schematic representation of a process. It is a particularly helpful tool for quality improvement projects when each step in a process is analyzed when searching for solutions to a problem. Typically, the following symbols are used:
Parallelogram: Input and output (start/end)
Arrow: Direction of flow
Diamond-shape: Conditional decision (Yes/No or True/False)
Circles: Connectors with diverging paths with multiple arrows coming in but only one going out.

146. B: Total Quality Management (TQM) is one philosophy of quality management that espouses a commitment to meeting the needs of the customers at all levels within an organization, promoting y continuous improvement and dedication to quality in all aspects of an organization. Outcomes should include increased customer satisfaction, productivity, and increased profits. Necessary elements:
Information regarding customer's needs and opinions.
Involvement of staff at all levels in decision making, goal setting, and problems solving.
Commitment of management to empowering staff and being accountable through active leadership and participation.
Institution of teamwork with incentives and rewards for accomplishments.

147. A: E&CFA is a combination of the flow chart and affinity diagram and is useful in root cause analysis:
List the name of the process/occurrence in a box on the right
List the steps in the process in boxes from right to left linked with arrows pointing to the process box on the right.
Under each event box, place an arrow pointing downward and list all possible factors contributing to the occurrence through repeatedly asking "Why?"
Discuss and reach group consensus about root causes to determine actions for performance improvement or to ensure the ability to replicate a process.

148. D: A Gantt chart is used for developing improvement projects to manage schedules and estimate time needed to complete tasks. It is a bar chart with a horizontal time scale that presents a visual representation of the beginning and end points of time when different steps in a process should be completed. Gantt charts are a component of project management software programs. The Gantt chart is usually created after initial brainstorming, and creation of a time line and action plans.

149. B: The source (nurse executive) decides what the message (content) to be sent is and the encoder (also the nurse executive) is the one who interprets the message in order to transmit it. In this case, the source of the information encoded it incorrectly so that it could

not be decoded by the patients. The channel is the method in which the message is transmitted.   The decoder is the person who interprets the message received. This may or may not be the receiver of the message.

150. C: In the Health Communication Model (Northouse and Northouse, 1992), **contexts** refers to the setting and the environmental conditions (including the number and types of people present). Different contexts affect communication in different ways. Another element is the 4 types of communication **relationships**: professional/professional, professional/client, professional/significant other, and client/significant other. The last element is **transactions**, which include verbal and non-verbal communication. These two forms of communication are considered equally important, especially if they are congruent.